CANCER STORIES

cancer stories
on Life and Suffering

David M. Gregory and Cynthia K. Russell

To Eleanor

With affection and admiration.

david

PUBLISHED FOR CARLETON UNIVERSITY
BY McGILL-QUEEN'S UNIVERSITY PRESS,
MONTREAL & KINGSTON, LONDON, ITHACA

Copyright © Carleton University Press, 1999

ISBN 0-88629-359-6 (cloth)
ISBN 0-88629-354-5 (paperback)

Printed and bound in Canada

Canadian Cataloguing in Publication Data

Gregory, David Michael, 1958-
    Cancer stories : on life and suffering

Includes bibliographical references.
ISBN 0-88629-359-6 (bound).—ISBN 0-88629-354-5 (pbk.)

    1. Cancer—Patients—Biography.   I. Russell, Cynthia K.
(Cynthia Kay), 1958-   II. Title.

RC265.5.G74 1999   362.1'96994'00922   C99-900927-3

Cover image: "Tree of Trees #2," by Kelly Clark©. Etching and collage on
paper, 1985, CARfac©Collective, 71.1 x 49.5 cm. Photographer: Earnest
Mayer
Cover design: David LeBlanc
Interior: Lynn's Desktop Publishing

This book has been published with the help of a grant from the Humanities
and Social Sciences Federation of Canada, using funds provided by the
Social Sciences and Humanities Research Council of Canada.

Canadä

McGill-Queen's University Press acknowledges the financial support of the
Government of Canada through the Book Publishing Industry Development
Program (BPIDP) for our publishing activities. We also acknowledge the sup-
port of the Canada Council for the Arts for our publishing program.

To those who journey with cancer
and teach us
about life and suffering.
*

In memory of Julia, Sarah,
Madeline, Kay, and John.

CONTENTS

ACKNOWLEDGMENTS

The authors thank Glennis Zilm, not only for her advice during the preliminary stages of this book, but for her faith.

We are indebted to the anonymous reviewers whose insightful comments encouraged us to examine critically the relationships among cancer, suffering, and science. Thanks to Frances Rooney for her skillful copyedit, and to Carleton University Press.

We also acknowledge Shirley Dyck who transcribed the voices and cancer journeys of Julia, Sarah, Madeline, Kay, and John.

I

CANCER: SUFFERING IN SILENCE

THROUGHOUT HISTORY diseases have defined eras. Tuberculosis, syphilis, leprosy, the Plague, smallpox, and polio all have their places in history. Some old illnesses are taking on new life, developing resistance to our medications and threatening to reassert their historical claims on the human body. HIV/AIDS, hantaviruses, and flesh-eating bacteria are the "new" contenders. Although textual, artistic, statistical, and media accounts of these old and new diseases offer us understanding of their power and impact, such accounts only become meaningful when a disease directly touches us. For most of us, these diseases will remain safely distanced from our lives.

A disease becomes known by the suffering it inflicts on those who live it, by its unique signature. This signature, which is etched in bodies, written into the "plots" of life stories, and woven into the social fabric of our times, is shaped primarily by two forces: pathophysiology, how disease occupies our bodies; and our lifeworld, how disease occupies our lives. Sometimes this occupation is brief and deadly. The Ebola virus, for example, takes hold of the body and ends life with devastating speed. In other instances, our bodies and our lives become overshadowed by chronic, debilitating illnesses.

Medicine focuses primarily on disease pathophysiology and pathoanatomy. The concern is with the natural history of disease. Physicians are interested in how a disease enters or develops in the body, what it does to the body, and how it can be prevented, or treated and controlled if prevention is not successful. Governments as well as public and private agencies spend billions of dollars worldwide in the quest for disease prevention and treatment. What is sought are general principles and universal scientific laws. This is a population- or epidemiological-based approach to knowing disease. Cancer is in the forefront of this quest for understanding.

Cancer: The Disease

Cancer is in reality several groups of diseases, each with its own diagnosis, treatment, and chances for control or cure. What is common to all cancers is the multiplication and uncontrollable growth of abnormal cells. Cells undergo mutation. They change and explode in a burst of misguided reproduction that results in excess tissue or tumours. These tumours can cause blockages or they can affect the ability of our cells and organs to function normally. This growth can also cause significant changes to our body chemistry. Our internal milieu becomes toxic. Eventually, such unregulated growth consumes our bodies. We waste away. Cancer's insatiable appetite takes what it needs to survive, growing while our bodies starve. Physicians call this state "cachexia." It is profound malnutrition. Accompanying this cellular growth and bodily starvation is fatigue. In the wake of such spectacular cellular activity, cancer produces a heavy, dense tiredness. As a consequence, sleep often loses its restorative properties.

There is another more treacherous aspect of cancer: it seeds. A primary tumour, the original cancer site, gives birth to secondary tumours and metastases. Some cancer cells, carried by blood or lymph fluids, float to other areas of the body. They settle, take root, and satellite tumours begin to grow in the body. These new sites also reproduce and grow at an alarming rate. Like their mother site, they consume the body's nutrients and can cause organ dysfunction. Other cancer cells may actually multiply in the body's fluids — the blood or lymph networks.

Cancer's propensity to seed makes treating this disease difficult. Original or primary tumours may be surgically removed from the body. One of the first questions people ask after surgical treatment is, "Did they get it all?" Progeny of the primary tumours are usually treated with chemotherapy or radiation. Radiation focuses on particular clumps of cells and kills them without surgery. Sometimes the entire body must undergo total or systemic treatment. Chemotherapy, for example, is used to kill cancer cells that may have seeded from a primary tumour elsewhere in the body. The choice of treatment depends on the kind of cancer and whether or nor it has spread from the original site.

Finally, cancer often hides in the body at least early on or initially. Physicians are greatly challenged to find cancer, both at the time of initial diagnosis and when trying to detect whether it has spread. Cancer takes up residence deep within our bodies, occupying flesh within flesh. It is found in the breast, liver, pancreas, colon, stomach, and other body parts. Living with cancer means living with fear, even after it is treated. Cancer may be concealed in tissue, virtually undetectable in the body.

Cancer has a long history. The Greeks named it "karkinos" (the crab). True to its name, this disease has slowly crept forward, gaining hold on the bodies and the lives of millions of people. The sheer volume of cancer has made this ancient disease of modern concern. Former U.S. President Nixon officially declared "war" on cancer in 1971. Since then there have been some victories. Survival rates have improved with respect to Hodgkin's Disease (a cancer of the lymph nodes), childhood leukaemia, and colon and rectal cancers. However, survival rates associated with solid tumours such as cancers of the breast, brain, pancreas, and liver remain relatively unchanged since Nixon's war cry. The war continues, but now there are many other battles; diseases competing not only for research dollars, but also for our compassion and understanding.

Changes in the Praxis of Science: Qualitative Research

Scientific or empirical knowing has demonstrated its awesome power in relation to disease. Modern medicine offers cures, treatments, and preventive measures for almost every disease known to humankind. Other ways of knowing, however, are integral to understanding disease, including: aesthetic, moral-ethical, and personal domains of knowledge.[1] As humans, our bodies and our lives are fundamentally and intimately whole. Focusing exclusively on the objective dimensions of disease (pathophysiology and body biology) ignores how disease is *lived* by persons. The human side of disease, the quality of life while living with disease, has only recently been accorded importance within the scientific community. Postmodern social scientists have discovered that the living of a disease is as important as its natural history. Disease is not simply a biological entity, but is constituted through social, cultural, and historical forces.

The human side of disease is captured through the qualitative paradigm. This paradigm, worldview, or way of "doing science" values personal and contextual domains of knowledge. Qualitative research methods give priority to persons and their disease journeys. This book uses narratives that are systematically analysed and synthesized personal stories. This is the research method that "gives voice" to the human side of cancer.

When held hostage by cancer it is not just our bodies, but our lives that become profoundly affected. Beyond biology and epidemiology, living with cancer is shaped by our individual life contexts. Who we are, our history and our dreams for the future, what we do for a living, our homelife, our family members and friends; these elements of the lifeworld influence how cancer is lived. It is in the specifics and details of a person's life that the human dimensions of cancer become apparent.

Suffering and Cancer

Suffering and cancer. These two words rarely appear together. There is a disturbing silence around suffering and cancer. Health care providers and cancer societies emphasize coping, hope, and "Looking Good-Feeling Good," while remaining relatively silent about suffering. Social scientists have traditionally known cancer through statistics and numerical indices. They have selectively and objectively applied tools and instruments to measure specific dimensions of the experience of cancer. This approach to science also keeps researchers at a safe distance from the human dimension of cancer. Missing from these perspectives and measures are the voices of people who are living with cancer.

Qualitative research challenges scientists to listen and "hear" the voices of their participants. Because language serves as the vehicle for social, cultural, historical, and contextual meanings embedded in words, the world of discourse makes known the suffering in the cancer experience. Qualitative research also challenges researchers to understand the cancer experience, and the suffering therein, in a more holistic manner.

Health care providers and researchers may minimize the suffering brought on by cancer. This malignant disease is spoken about in the most benign of terms. Cancer-as-suffering is described by words or phrases stripped of emotion. People living with cancer are said to experience "distress," "problems," "pain," "side effects of treatment," "changes in body image," and "psychosocial concerns." The realities of cancer are lived by different words. The worlds of those who live with and die from cancer are filled with great emotion and suffering.

It is only recently that many of the silences concerning cancer have been broken. People in Canada and the United States are whispering less and talking more. Cancer, the disease, is out in the open. It is the topic of television talk shows, science documentaries, art work, and self-help books. There remains, however, a significant silence in relation to people who are living with and dying from cancer.

Why should we be concerned about suffering and cancer? Silence may actually increase the suffering experienced by people living with this disease. People can be consumed twice over: by cancer and by their suffering. Acknowledging the suffering in cancer, talking about it, and validating it, can help people live more fully. Such understanding may assist people to better prepare for their cancer journeys. Knowing that others suffer also validates our own suffering. When we are silent about the realities endured by those who live with cancer, we diminish their plight.

The Illness Experience as a Source of Suffering

Suffering has traditionally been the concern of the religious. Within societies, religions have assumed responsibility for helping people come to terms with suffering. Western religions typically frame suffering as a "problem" (e.g., the problem of theodicy: How could a good and loving God permit His people to suffer), while Eastern religions generally understand suffering as "mystery." Regardless of perspective, the purpose of religions is to offer comfort to the sufferer, his or her family, and society in general. Religions provide explanations and attempt to make sense of suffering. They try to help us understand this perplexing human condition.

Over the centuries, medicine gradually embraced the tenets of science and moved away from the mysticism, magic, and myth that were often associated with religious or metaphysical beliefs. Science offered physicians and society a belief system based on objectivity and fact. There was no place for suffering within this new belief system where people were understood through a mechanical metaphor: the machine. Just as a functional machine can be understood through dissecting it into its component parts, so persons became reduced and known through their component parts — cells, organs, and systems. Suffering, when acknowledged, was equated to pain rooted in the body.

There is one branch of biomedicine that acknowledges suffering. Palliative care recognizes the concept of "total pain." Effective palliative care entails exploring pain in relation to a person's physical, emotional, social, cultural, and spiritual dimensions. That stated, there remains an impulse within the scientific community to frame suffering as a physiologically based phenomenon.[2] Others [3] view this understanding as the medicalization of suffering whereby "the quest to *control* [emphasis added] suffering transforms a profoundly complex human experience into essentially a physical condition amenable to treatment"(18).

Only in the last few years have physicians, nurses, and allied health workers been reminded that suffering is central to the illness experience. Travelbee,[4] Kleinman,[5] and Cassell[6] have drawn people's suffering to our attention. Their work identifies that bodies are cured, but healing involves persons and their suffering experiences. Sick people suffer. Suffering is something that persons, and not just bodies, experience.

Knowing Suffering through Cancer

Everyone in the world suffers, not only people with cancer. Paradoxically, this universal experience occurs at the most intimate level of our being. "While women and men feel anguish and die in the millions, suffering the same accidents, famines, diseases, plagues and wars, each of their lives merits a singular story"(16).[7] It is on this last point that the purpose of this book unfolds. Five people — Julia, Sarah, Madeline, Kay, and John — who died of cancer, who suffered a common disease and a common fate, share their unique stories. Each of their lives and deaths merits a singular story. And thus, the often untold suffering encountered while living with cancer and dying from cancer is revealed in these five stories or narratives.

This book was written for several reasons. Giving "voice" to those who did not survive their cancer was paramount. In contrast, cancer survivors freely tell their tales of overcoming adversity and "beating cancer." These are often heroic and inspirational stories. They are positive accounts and uplifting testimonials of the human spirit. They are pleasant reading and leave us feeling good. These stories are *de rigueur* in a society obsessed with self-help manuals to life and living. Dying of cancer is replete with failure: the concomitant failures of medicine, our bodies, and the will to "beat" this disease.

Hope is the central message offered by cancer survivors. "I beat cancer and so can you!" Yet, what about the millions of people who do not survive cancer? What can be said about them? Theirs is the other, the silent, reality. People who do not survive cancer also have stories, but of a different kind. Theirs are accounts of living and dying with a consumptive disease. The narratives in this book permit the reader to journey with five people as they travel along their cancer paths. These are difficult journeys, but worth the effort. These people welcome us as co-journeyers to the private struggles and intimate details of their lives.

The five narratives in this book are brutally honest accounts. While the stories share some things in common, they are five different journeys. Each is a chronicle of the often untold suffering encountered with cancer. The stories are raw and real accounts of the lived experience of cancer.

Lessons Learned and the "Gifts" Offered

People who die of cancer have much to share with others. Unlike survivors, the hope offered by these five people is not limited to "beating cancer." Rather, the hope in the five narratives relates to living as fully as possible despite the horrors brought by cancer. This hope also speaks of the need for love and meaningful relationships in life. Living fully with advanced cancer means understanding and accepting that suffering can be part of this journey.

Lessons learned are presented as "gifts" at the conclusion of each of the five narratives. Some of the lessons are emotionally painful. Others are joyful. Deeply sorrowful moments merge with life-affirming experiences. By accompanying Julia, Sarah, Madeline, Kay, and John on their cancer paths, we come to know their experiences, their suffering, joy, and pain, and what happened to them. Learning from them teaches us about the realities of advanced cancer. This is practical knowledge embedded in experience. Persons living with and dying from cancer develop intimate understanding of their disease. Heidegger,[8] Gadamer,[9] and Benner[10] have long recognized the value of knowledge embedded in experience. It is knowledge arising from the personal, aesthetic, and moral-ethical domains of persons' lives which is revealed at the end of each narrative. These discoveries are possible through the conduct of qualitative research.

A Word of Advice to the Reader

This book is different from other books about cancer. The people whose stories are presented do not survive. They all die. The chapters preceding the narratives provide important information. We recommend that you read these first few chapters before embarking on the cancer journeys.

Chapter two, "Paths of Science," gives technical and statistical information about breast cancer, ovarian cancer, and malignant melanoma. Julia, Sarah, and Madeline died of breast cancer, Kay of ovarian cancer, John from malignant melanoma. Brief information about the treatment of these cancers is also highlighted. This chapter demonstrates the distance between the scientific language and the lived experience of cancer. Reading about cancer from a scientific perspective and then reading how each person lived with the reality of their cancer — the tests, treatments, and side effects of chemotherapy — provides a stark contrast between the science and humanity of cancer.

Background information as to "how" the narratives were written is outlined in chapter three. More importantly, it prepares you for the difficult stories that follow. You are introduced to the gifts these five people offer. Reading this chapter before the narratives will permit you to see not only the suffering, but the wisdom of experience captured in the five narratives.

Chapters four to eight are the stories or narratives proper. These are the accounts as told by Julia, Sarah, Madeline, Kay, and John. The narratives are written so that you are gradually drawn into their lives. You will get to know them. Page by page you will discover the impact of cancer on their lives.

The last chapter contains a discussion concerning life and suffering. What can be said about suffering in light of these five narratives, of the five lives that succumbed to cancer? At the end of the book you will have a better understanding of the nature of suffering related to cancer. You will come to know what dimensions of the cancer experience contribute to our suffering and how some of these can be managed or endured. The narratives reveal that not all suffering can be treated with a pill, a tonic, or a counselling session. You will also discover how some people were able to transcend or come to terms with their suffering. Finally, the experiential knowledge uncovered in each of the narratives can prepare us to live more fully with advanced cancer, should cancer enter our lives or the lives of those we love.

2

CANCER PATHS: THE SCIENCE

cancer (kan'ser) [G. karkinos, crab] An imprecise term used to describe an estimated 200 different kinds of malignant neoplasms, marked by uncontrolled growth and the spread of abnormal cells. Cancers may be lethal by invading adjacent normal tissues or by spread (metastasis) to sites distant from the place of origin. Cancers that arise in epithelial tissues are called carcinomas; from mesenchymal tissues, sarcomas. Leukemias are also considered malignant growths.

— Taber's Cyclopedic Medical Dictionary

INFORMATION IN THIS CHAPTER is technical in nature. Included are statistics for breast cancer, ovarian cancer, and malignant melanoma. Risk factors (behaviours or conditions that promote the development of cancer) and general treatment protocols for these cancers are also outlined. The distance between cancer pathophysiology and living with cancer as it unfolds in the lives of people, becomes evident when this chapter is contrasted with the narratives. Science, with its passion for the cellular behaviour of cancer, remains disembodied from the lives of persons living with cancer. Science easily overpowers subjective accounts of cancer and therefore, it has been placed in this chapter, separate from the cancer stories.

BREAST CANCER

The Statistics

Breast cancer is a major source of suffering and death for North American women. Statistics associated with this disease are staggering. The number of new cases of breast cancer has steadily increased at a rate of one to two percent per year since the 1960s.[11] The National Cancer Institute estimated that 18,700 Canadian women were diagnosed with breast cancer in 1999.[12] In 1995, 17,700 Canadian women[13] and over 180,000 American women[14] were diagnosed with breast cancer. In Canada, over 5,400 women will have lost their lives to this disease in 1999. Approximately 46,000 American women died of breast cancer during 1995. Imagine a city of 50,000 people — this is how many women died of breast cancer in Canada and the United States during the past 12 months. It is difficult to fathom these numbers. On average, five new cases of breast cancer are diagnosed and at least one woman dies of breast cancer every 15 minutes in the United States.[15] Beyond the statistics, breast cancer causes immense suffering — for women, their partners, their families, and their friends.

Approximately a decade ago, in 1991, the Canadian and American Cancer Societies estimated that the average woman's risk for developing breast cancer was one in nine. Currently, the chances are very good that one woman out of eight will develop breast cancer during her lifetime. That more women are now being diagnosed with breast cancer than ever before may be partly related to improved detection of breast cancer through mammography. Women with breast cancer are being diagnosed sooner in the course of their disease. Mammography — a screening X-ray of the breast — detects small cancerous lumps in the breast before they can be felt by a woman. Outside of this technology, nearly 90 percent of all breast lumps are discovered by women or their partners. The lump is found most often in the upper outer section of the breast.[16]

The number of Canadian women dying of breast cancer decreased by 0.1 percent between 1983 and 1992. The number of American women dying from breast cancer declined by 4.7 percent between 1989 and 1992, the largest such short-term decline in the United States for this disease since 1950. This decline may have been related to early detection through screening, improved treatment, or changes in risk or protective factors. More women in the United States and Canada will die of lung cancer, but cancer of the breast is the leading cause of cancer death in women aged 20 to 49. Lung cancer tends to be a disease of "older" women, whereas breast cancer claims the lives of younger women.

There is no single known cause of breast cancer. Risk factors, characteristics that appear to increase the probability of a woman developing breast cancer, include:[17]

- gender;
- age (the incidence of breast cancer increases with age);

- personal history (a previous breast cancer diagnosis increases a woman's risk for developing a second breast cancer in the opposite breast);
- family history of cancer (women with a family history of breast cancer in a first-degree relative [mother, sister, or daughter] have a risk that is two to three times higher than the general population);
- genetics (there may be a role in genetic transmission of tumour suppression genes);
- early menarche (before the age of 12) and late menopause (after the age of 50);
- reproductive history (having no children or the first full-term pregnancy after the age of 30);
- benign breast disease;
- obesity (postmenopausal women) and dietary fat.

Women diagnosed with breast cancer may or may not have any of these risk factors. It is likely that breast cancer develops as a consequence of many different factors that vary from woman to woman.

Treating Breast Cancer

The treatment of breast cancer is complex and evolving. Treatment approaches include various combinations of surgery, radiation, chemotherapy, and hormonal therapy. Physicians consider several factors when determining the treatment of choice for a specific woman: the stage of the cancer, the location of the lump, the age of the woman and her choice regarding preservation of her breast, for example. The goal of treatment is to provide women with the best possible chance of survival and quality of living. Cancer that is small in size and is contained within the breast is at an early stage. The prognosis or treatment outcome of early stage breast cancer is better than cancer diagnosed at a later stage. In late stage cancer — metastatic cancer — the lump is larger and the cancer has spread to other parts of the body. The most effective combinations of treatment approaches (for example, surgery and chemotherapy) are being researched by scientists all over the world.

The standard treatment approach for small tumours is breast-saving surgery followed by 5 to 7 weeks of postoperative radiation.[18] It is only in the last 15 years that breast saving techniques have been used in the treatment of breast cancer. A common procedure is the lumpectomy. The cancer tumour (lump) is surgically removed; the rest of the breast is left intact. Another type of breast-saving surgery is the partial mastectomy. In addition to the removal of the cancerous lump, some normal breast tissue surrounding the lump is also cut away. Sometimes, depending on the stage of the breast cancer and the location of the tumour, it is necessary to remove the entire breast. This operation is called a simple (total) mastectomy. The whole breast is surgically cut away, but chest muscles and lymph nodes are left in place. For many years, the modified radical mastectomy was the standard surgical procedure for breast cancer regardless of stage. During a modified radical mastectomy, the total breast is removed along with the axillary lymph nodes and the lining of the chest muscle.

Often during a partial mastectomy, the surgeon will remove 5 to 10 lymph nodes in the underarm area. This is called axillary node dissection. Lymph nodes are small bean-like structures that fight bacteria, viruses and cancer cells in the blood. There are approximately 30 to 40 lymph nodes in the underarm area. The nodes are examined by a pathologist for the presence of cancer; they are viewed under a microscope to see whether cancer has spread beyond the breast. If cancer is present in the lymph nodes, it is called "node positive." This usually means that chemotherapy, drugs that kill cancer cells, will be required. Knowing whether the nodes are positive or negative helps the oncologist determine the stage of the cancer and the required treatment after surgery; chemotherapy, radiation, or hormone therapy. Whether axillary (underarm) lymph nodes are positive or negative is considered to be the most important prognostic factor for breast cancer patients.[19] Survival rates tend to decrease as the number of positive nodes increase. But while women who have positive nodes are more likely than those with negative nodes to have a recurrence of breast cancer, breast cancer recurs in about one-third of women who are node-negative.

Adjuvant therapy — treatment in addition to surgery — is usually started within 4 to 12 weeks after surgery. The purpose of adjuvant therapy is to kill any cancer cells that have spread beyond the original tumour site. After a lumpectomy or a partial mastectomy, radiation to the breast is used to prevent the recurrence of cancer. Radiation uses high energy X-rays to kill cancer cells and shrink tumours. Adjuvant chemotherapy is also recommended after surgery when there is a chance that cancer cells have spread beyond the breast. Combinations of drugs are usually taken intravenously or orally to poison the cancer cells which reproduce or grow rapidly. Chemotherapy also kills fast-growing cells throughout the body. Fast-growing cells include breast cancer cells along with other cells such as hair follicles and bone-marrow cells which produce red and white blood cells for the body. This is why women who undergo chemotherapy treatments typically lose their hair and experience nausea, diarrhea, or sores in their mouths. Sometimes chemotherapy has to be stopped because it causes the levels of white blood cells to drop dangerously low; with low levels of white blood cells, a person cannot "fight off" infections.

Like chemotherapy, hormone therapy may be used to treat breast cancer, especially when there is a chance that cancer cells have spread beyond the breast. Every situation of breast cancer is different and, consequently, treatments will vary from woman to woman.

Living with Breast Cancer

Dedicated physicians and researchers, concerned with developing more sensitive diagnostic tests and effective treatments for breast cancer, walk alongside women on their breast cancer paths. The voices of physicians and scientists are heard at scientific conferences and in published research papers. The language of scientists and physicians is technical in nature and focuses on the causes of cancer, chromosomes, diagnostic procedures, and clinical research trials. This is the voice of science.

The voices of women who walk on breast cancer paths are difficult to hear amid the sounds of science. Beyond science — undergoing the diagnostic tests, living through the treatments, and living with breast cancer — womens' voices speak a different reality, a different language. Over 200,000 women in Canada and the United States will be diagnosed with breast cancer this year. Each woman, while sharing common experiences related to breast cancer and its treatment, has her own story to tell, her own path to proceed along.

The voices of women who do not survive breast cancer are rarely heard. In this book three women — Julia, Sarah, and Madeline — share their breast cancer stories and their journeys. Documenting their paths and journeys provides us with a sense of what it is really like to live with, and die from, breast cancer. Silenced by death, their struggles and sorrows are lost to cancer and history. And yet their voices call out to other women, "*I was diagnosed and treated for breast cancer. I lived with and died from breast cancer. This is what happened to me!*" These women live on through their stories and offer the reader their experiences with breast cancer.

OVARIAN CANCER

The Statistics

Among Canadian women, incidence and death rates for ovarian cancer have continued to decline steadily. The number of new cases of ovarian cancer decreased by 1.7 percent between 1983 and 1990. Similarly, the number of Canadian women dying of this cancer fell by 0.9 percent during this same time period.[20] In 1999, the estimated incidence for ovarian cancer was 14 women per 100,000 population. Approximately 2,600 Canadian women were diagnosed with ovarian cancer and, like their American sisters, more than half of the women with a diagnosis of ovarian cancer (1,500) will have died in 1999.[21] Ovarian cancer constituted approximately 4 percent of all new cancer cases among Canadian women and 4.8 percent of all cancer deaths were attributed to ovarian cancer during this same year.

In 1995, ovarian cancer constituted 5 percent of all newly diagnosed cancers among American women (breast cancer, in comparison, was the most frequently occurring cancer site, comprising 32 percent of all new cancers).[22] It was estimated that 26,600 American women were diagnosed with ovarian cancer and more than 14,000 women died of ovarian cancer in 1995. Cancer of the ovary was the leading cause of death in terms of gynecological cancers, which include cancers of the uterus and the cervix.[23] Ovarian cancer was the fifth leading cause of death among American women aged 35 to 54, and the fourth most commonly reported cause of cancer death among women aged 55 to 74.[24] When diagnosed early, when cancer is limited to the ovary, the five-year survival rate for White women is high — approximately 90 percent.[25] For Black American women, however, the rate is lower, at 85 percent. Unfortunately, ovarian cancer is not generally diagnosed early, as 77 percent of women have advanced ovarian cancer at the time of diagnosis.

The Nature of Ovarian Cancer

The two ovaries are the female reproductive organs that contain ova (eggs). Ovaries release the female hormone estrogen. Estrogen helps support pregnancy and contributes to female sex characteristics (for example, the development of breasts and the establishment of menstruation). The ovaries are made up of cells. When these cells grow abnormally, a tissue mass or tumour forms. These tumours can be benign or malignant (cancer).

There are three basic types of ovarian cancer: epithelial cell, germ cell, and stromal cell.[26] About 90 percent of all ovarian cancer develops from the cells that line the surface of the ovaries; these cancers are called epithelial cell tumours. Epithelial tumours are most frequently found in women aged 40 to 65 years of age and account for 85 percent of all ovarian malignancies diagnosed in the United States.[27] Ovarian cancer can also arise from the germ or egg cells found in the ovary as well as from stromal cells which make up the ovarian structures. The epithelial cell type of ovarian cancer can spread to the other ovary, the uterus, fallopian tubes, bladder, rectum, and peritoneum (lining of the abdomen). Malignant cells are shed and float throughout the peritoneal cavity. These cells plant themselves and, unlike most other cancers, grow outward rather than invading deeper layers of tissue. This type of ovarian cancer also tends to produce fluid in the abdomen and can cause the bowels to adhere. Ovarian cancer arising from germ cells affects younger women; it is very rare and responds well to treatment. Ovarian cancer arising from the stromal cells is also very rare. It occurs, however, in women of any age and tends to respond less well to treatment.

Although the risks must be considered, the use of oral contraceptives may reduce the chances of ovarian cancer. Ovarian cancer is "silent" in the early stages and this is why most women have metastases at the time of their diagnosis. A recently developed blood test may detect the presence of ovarian cancer and thus enable early treatment. Protective factors against ovarian cancer include more than one full-term pregnancy and breast feeding. A possible protective factor is tubal ligation. The risk of women developing ovarian cancer over a lifetime increases with the number of first-degree family members (mothers, sisters, and daughters) diagnosed with this disease.

The early signs and symptoms of ovarian cancer include vague and persistent digestive disturbances such as heartburn, indigestion, weight loss, nausea, and feeling full right after commencing to eat. If ovarian cancer remains undetected and untreated, other symptoms appear. The most common one is an enlarged abdomen. Swelling is caused by a collection of fluid in the abdomen and is linked to the presence of ovarian cancer cells. Sometimes this swelling is related to the tumour itself or to fluid produced by the tumour. Abnormal vaginal bleeding may also occur.

Treating Ovarian Cancer

Several diagnostic techniques are used to confirm the presence of cancer and to determine whether or not it has spread. These may include specialized X-rays, CT scan (computerized tomography, which provides detailed pictures of internal organs and tissues), ultrasound tests (a test where high frequency sound waves are "bounced" against tissues to "see" if a tumour or mass is present), and blood tests. During an exploratory laparotomy, the inside of the abdomen is inspected by inserting a little scope or camera through an incision near the belly button. This device is also used to take tissue samples to determine whether a mass is cancerous.

Ovarian cancer is generally treated by a combination of surgery, radiation, and chemotherapy. Surgery typically entails removal of one or both of the ovaries. Frequently, the uterus (the womb) and fallopian tubes (tubes leading from the ovaries to the uterus down which the woman's egg passes each month as part of the menstrual cycle) are taken out as a preventive measure or because cancer cells have spread to these structures. The extent of surgery depends upon the type of cancer found and how much it has spread.

Following surgery, chemotherapy or radiation is often used to destroy any remaining cancer cells. Radiation is usually initiated to treat women in the early stages of ovarian cancer. For women with high risk, early stage epithelial ovarian tumours, chemotherapy has resulted in improved response rates and increased disease-free survival.[28] If ovarian cancer is detected and treated while the tumour is confined to the ovaries, most women are alive and active five years later. If the tumour has spread to other organs in the pelvic area, the chances of a cure are not so good.

Living with Ovarian Cancer

More than 28,000 Canadian and American women were diagnosed and began their journeys with ovarian cancer in 1995.[29] One woman's story is included in this book. Kay was not one of the fortunate women diagnosed with localized ovarian cancer. Hers had metastasized far beyond both her ovaries by the time she was diagnosed. Kay's story is ultimately tragic. It is a life and death account of a mother who tries to survive ovarian cancer, who struggles against the statistical odds of advanced cancer. Kay's voice is one of more than the approximately

15,000 Canadian and American women who lose their lives to ovarian cancer each year.[30]

The Statistics

When discovered early, most types of skin cancer are treatable. Malignant melanoma — a specific kind of skin cancer — occurs in younger age groups. In Canada, just over 3,500 people were diagnosed with malignant melanoma in 1999 and this disease claimed an estimated 770 lives.[31] As in the United States, malignant melanoma will account for just over 2 percent of all new cancers in men and 2.5 percent of all new cancers in women. The percentage of deaths related to melanoma among Canadian men and women paralleled that of the United States. The death rate for melanoma among men is rising at 1.9 percent per year. Among women, the yearly number of deaths attributed to melanoma has decreased by 1 percent. The five-year survival rate for men is much lower (57 percent) than that of women (77 percent). In 1995, just over 34,000 Americans[32] were diagnosed with melanoma. In the same year, approximately 7,200 Americans died of this disease.[33]

Melanoma accounted for 3 percent of newly diagnosed cancer cases and was the cause of 2 percent of all cancer deaths in men and 1 percent of all cancer deaths in women. The relative five-year survival rate is 93 percent when melanoma has not spread beyond the local site — the place where the cancer started to grow. Once melanoma moves beyond the local site, however, survival rates drop dramatically: to 58 percent when it spreads just beyond the original site, and 14 percent when it spreads to distant parts of the body.[34]

There are two major kinds of skin cancer: nonmelanoma and malignant melanoma. Basal cell and squamous cell carcinomas (cancers) are nonmelanomas. More than 93 percent of all skin cancers are from the nonmelanoma group.[35] Malignant melanoma is cancer that is found in the cells that give colour to the skin (melanocytes). Melanocytes contain melanin, the substance which colours skin. Malignant melanoma is becoming more common and it is affecting younger people. Malignant melanoma is typically a cancer of fair-skinned people. Among men, melanoma is most often found along the upper back and the trunk. Common sites for women to develop melanoma include the back and the legs. Dark-skinned people, among whom this is a rare disease, develop melanoma on the palms of the hands, soles of the feet, nailbeds, fingers, and toes.

There are several risk factors associated with developing malignant melanoma.[36] Exposure to the sun and where one lives in relation to the equator are two of the most important contributors to the onset of melanoma. Sustaining severe sunburns, particularly during childhood and adolescence, increases the risk of this cancer later in life. People who burn easily, who do not tan, are also at risk. For example, people of fair complexion or those persons with blonde or red hair experience higher cancer rates because they have less melanin, the substance that filters out the sun's rays. Although tanning, the skin's response to ultraviolet light, is a protective reaction to prevent further injury to the skin, it does not prevent skin cancer. A family history of this disease is also considered a risk factor. Men and women who spend long hours in the sun — farmers, people who fish, sailors, and other outdoor workers — have an increased risk of developing this type of skin cancer.

The primary risk factor associated with skin cancer is solar exposure. Ultraviolet radiation penetrates the skin causing changes in blood vessels and premature aging of the skin; it is associated with skin cancer. Measures that reduce sun damage to the skin include using sun screens with sun protection factor (SPF) ratings of 15 or higher; protecting children from sunburns; avoiding intense sunlight between 10:00 A.M. and 3:00 P.M. since ultraviolet radiation is greatest at this time; avoiding sunlamps and tanning parlours; and wearing protective clothing such as hats and long-sleeved shirts. The level of ultraviolet light is higher now than it was 50 years ago; a reduction of ozone in the earth's atmosphere permits higher levels of ultraviolet light to reach the earth's surface.

Early detection and treatment of malignant melanoma are important to survival. Melanoma can spread quickly to other parts of the body through the lymph system or through the blood. Skin that becomes scaly or oozes, and moles or dark growths that bleed need medical attention. Early signs of malignant melanoma also include a change in colour or size of a mole or dark patch of skin; a spread of the darkened area beyond the normal border; a change in sensation, itchiness, tenderness or pain; or the development of a lump.[37]

Treating Malignant Melanoma

When malignant melanoma is suspected, a skin biopsy is taken. The entire growth, along with some of the nearby skin tissue is removed and examined under a microscope. A variety of laboratory tests are also usually conducted. For example, a blood profile, liver enzyme tests, urine analysis, and a chest X-ray. These tests provide a physician with additional information about whether the melanoma has metastasized.

The prognosis or outcome is based on how deeply the melanoma has grown and the thickness of the tumour itself. Surgery is the primary treatment. A wide excision or cut is made, removing the cancer and a swath of normal tissue. Lymph nodes near the cancer site are sometimes removed, depending on the size of the malignant melanoma. Chemotherapy drugs are also used to treat melanoma. However, melanoma does not usually respond to radiation treatments in terms of halting the disease. Radiation, to relieve discomfort or pain associated from metastasis (spread of cancer) to the bone, brain, and other organs, is often helpful to many people.

Living with Malignant Melanoma

John, one of approximately 8,000 Canadians and Americans who died of malignant melanoma this year, gives voice to the consumptive nature of this cancer. We are privy to his suffering, his struggles, and ultimately his death on this very difficult cancer path. Melanoma was diagnosed on the sole of John's right foot. He underwent surgery, chemotherapy, and palliative radiation. John's story is a tragic account of the consequences of advanced malignant melanoma.

Cancer, understood through the voice of science, is about statistics, research, diagnosis and treatment. Julia, Sarah, Madeline, Kay, and John tell us about the human experience of cancer. It is through their journeys that we come to understand how this disease enters not only bodies but lives.

Cancer is much more than cells. The narratives are much more than maudlin accounts of terminal illness; they are the stories behind the statistics. We learn how five people lived the best they could with cancer. We also come to know how personhood is preserved in the face of this consumptive disease.

3

THE CANCER STORIES

ALL DISEASES ARE REPLETE with suffering. HIV/AIDS, heart and kidney failure, cancer, and multiple sclerosis are examples of chronic and debilitating diseases which generate suffering within our lives. What these diseases share in common is how they gradually erode and undermine "the self." They assault who we are physically, psychologically, spiritually, and socially. We struggle to protect ourselves in the face of these consumptive onslaughts. Cancer, in this book, is the lens through which suffering is examined.

The intent of these cancer stories is not to fuel the fears that many already hold about cancer. Yes, the stories in this book are about people who lived with and died from cancer. Living with any debilitating disease, however, means trying to relocate it to the background of one's life, while simultaneously concentrating on the foreground and the living that takes place there. Cancer, given its natural history and the way it occupies our bodies, often moves from the background, takes over central aspects of life, and then recedes to the periphery. This is the rhythm of cancer. Periods of respite eventually become less frequent and finally disappear.

Four women and one man permitted one of the researchers (Gregory) to journey with them on their cancer paths over a period of up to six months. Three of the women — Julia, Sarah, and Madeline — were diagnosed and treated for breast cancer. Kay was treated for ovarian cancer. John's cancer, malignant melanoma, was detected in the sole of his foot. The name, diagnosis, age, and occupation of these five people are listed in Table 1. The average age of the participants was 48 years; these were people in the prime of their lives.

Table 1. THE PEOPLE WHO LIVED WITH AND DIED FROM CANCER*

Person	Diagnosis	Age	Occupation
Julia	breast cancer	51	nurse
Sarah	breast cancer	37	secretary
Madeline	breast cancer	41	cashier
Kay	ovarian cancer	50	mother
John	malignant melanoma	59	salesman

* To protect the identities of these five people and their family members, names have been changed along with some of the details concerning their lives.

Each person was interviewed once a week for up to six months to fathom the suffering in his or her life. The purpose of the unstructured interviews was twofold; people reflected upon their lives through a process of life review, and they identified the good and bad things that happened to them on a weekly basis. Accompanying those who were living with cancer as they journeyed provided a window to their life worlds. Although personal worlds can never be known completely, the five cancer narratives are intimate accounts, over time, of what it is like to live with and die from cancer.

The 89 "official" interviews were tape recorded and then transcribed verbatim. In addition to being interviewed, the participants were accompanied to places where they engaged in life activities: a flea market, cancer clinics, church services, a cemetery, restaurants, grocery stores, parks, and bookstores. Field observations were written down in a notebook by the researcher concerning these visits. The typed interviews and the written fieldnotes generated over 2,000 pages of textual data.

Construction of the Narratives

Each person's set of interviews, as captured on tape and in the typed interviews, was written up as a story. The substance of the narrative was important; those events that were spoken about by the person. In addition to "what" was said, the "how" of the telling was also significant. Meanings are conveyed in how people talk about what is happening to them. The emotions, delight, and grief in these people's voices are noted in the narratives.

The narratives were constructed one at a time and in the order in which the people were encountered: Julia, Sarah, Madeline, Kay, and

John. After the interviews were typed up, the interviewer read them from beginning to end. Then each interview was reread and key events or episodes identified. These episodes, both positive and negative, were noted in the margins of the transcripts. The full set of interviews and observations for each person was then analysed. For example, all of John's 17 interviews and 22 observation periods were read through and the key events noted. The researcher then wove the events together in a narrative. Episodes or events were organized according to their timing during the cancer journey. Response to a cancer diagnosis, for example, was placed before a response to a treatment, even though the participants might disclose information about the treatment before that about their diagnosis. While the participants conveyed meaning to their experiences and shared the details of their lives, the researchers later imposed temporal ordering on their narrations.

Captured in the interviews are the journeys of these five people as they lived with cancer. The question, "What happened to you this week?" was most often answered without pause over the course of one to two hours. Over time, as trust developed between the researcher and the person living with cancer, these interviews became an outpouring of the heart and soul.

The interviews took place in the homes of the participants, where they felt safe and secure. Kay was an exception. She was interviewed in her beautiful "purple garden" during the summer months. With the arrival of fall and eventually winter, the interviews were held in the researcher's car. The car heater offered some warmth during these sessions. Kay did not want anyone in her home. She felt that the "smell of cancer" was detectable throughout her house. From Kay's perspective, cancer filled her home as it did her body and her life.

These five narratives give voice to those who did not survive their cancer. Reading their stories permits us to get close to these people's lives and their experiences with this disease. The people who were interviewed wanted their stories shared with others. Julia, Sarah, and Madeline — the women with breast cancer — were particularly vocal about sharing their experiences with other women. They wanted people living with cancer, their families, and their friends, to know what happened so that they could help others. They wanted their encounters with cancer to matter.

Cancer is not an automatic death sentence. Not every woman diagnosed with breast cancer will die. Julia, Sarah, and Madeline did. Nor will every woman diagnosed with ovarian cancer die. Kay did.

Malignant melanoma is treatable if discovered and treated early. John, however, died from this disease.

Untold Suffering: Courage of the Human Spirit

Courage is central to these stories. It took courage on the part of Julia, Sarah, Madeline, Kay, and John to allow themselves to be accompanied on their cancer journeys, to reveal intimate moments, to lay bare their vulnerability, their fondest hopes, their greatest fears.

Courage is also required of the reader. Reading about the lives and deaths of these five people is not easy. The reading is made more difficult given the details of the lives captured in the narratives. As we read their stories, we become attached to the narrators. Our initial encounters are with strangers: people living with cancer. As the stories unfold, however, we begin to understand these strangers as real people whose lives intersected with a consumptive disease. We begin to relate to Julia, Sarah, and Madeline, whose breasts were surgically removed. We feel for Kay, a mother who tried to survive ovarian cancer. We come to know the terrible aloneness of John as he journeyed with malignant melanoma.

And so it is through courage, and with courage, that the cancer narratives follow.

4

JULIA

LIVING IN A STATE OF UNCERTAINTY:
BREAST CANCER

JULIA'S IS THE STORY OF A WOMAN who completes a course of treatment for breast cancer and then "waits out" her disease. Her suffering takes root in the constant monitoring of an unpredictable disease. Cancer places Julia in a difficult landscape. Julia's state is liminal; not cured, yet not in active treatment, she is located somewhere between these two realities. The following account is Julia's narrative, her story, her experience with cancer. Dimensions of her life are explored: her early history, the presence of cancer in her family, and Julia's beliefs about cancer. Finally, Julia invites us to travel along her cancer path. Uncertainty and the dread of recurrence are found on this path. Despite her diagnosis, Julia lives with breast cancer and engages life.

Julia's short, sandy brown hair is evidence of recent chemotherapy treatments and the toll exacted on her body. Glasses rest on her friendly, open face. She wears comfortable clothes; fleece and cotton sweats. She is also comfortable with herself, with her stage in life, who she is and what she has accomplished. Water is Julia's medium, her element. Enveloping and embracing her, it buoys her spirit. Swimming suspends Julia from the burden of her disease. In water, Julia forgets cancer and the heavy weight of her mastectomy. Julia swims a mile to celebrate her fifty-first birthday.

The Early Years

Julia was born in a small Missouri town; the second born child of working class parents. Like the Mississippi River flowing past their home, Julia's family was constantly on the move. Her father enlisted in the army shortly after her birth.

During the war she [mother] went and lived at some of the different army
bases and so one of the things my mom always took great pride in was the
fact that I had travelled like 25,000 miles by the time I was one year old.

The women in Julia's family work outside the home and she is
no exception. Julia states with pride that she is the first person in her
family to attend and complete college. While studying nursing, Julia
met and married Michael. The Great Plains called out to the young
couple and they responded by establishing a home and then a family
in the mid-western United States.

Julia speaks of coming from a dysfunctional family; a family thick
with conflict. Her father quit the military and then moved from job
to job, from problem to problem. Julia remembers something about
an extramarital affair involving her mother or possibly her father. A
fuzzy recollection, it is buried in the innocence of childhood memory.
Her mother committed suicide in 1972. Julia's father suffers from
Alzheimer's disease. He is cared for in a nearby nursing home. Julia's
older sister Angela has a history of failed marriages, financial difficulties, and legal problems.

Julia and Michael enjoy birding, dining out, and each other's company. They are friends as well as lovers. Well educated and earning dual
incomes, they live in a middle class neighbourhood. Their house is
spacious and furnished without extravagance. Julia's tastes reflect mid-
western sensibility; minimalism in concert with the flat, treeless land
and the forever sky. Her son and two daughters left home several years
ago and are now raising families of their own. Julia revels in being
a grandmother. Her two grandchildren are a source of great joy and
comfort, and Julia takes every opportunity to look after them. She
treasures them. She spoils them. She loves them dearly.

Julia works as a nurse in a community hospital. A bright, energetic
woman, Julia is widely read and knowledgeable about medical-surgical
nursing. She has also cared for people with cancer.

Cancer in the Family

Only Julia has cancer. With no known history of breast cancer, she
accepts responsibility for contributing cancer to the future generations
of women in her family. Her cancer diagnosis heralds a family legacy.

There's no history of cancer. I do genealogy as a hobby, so I know what they
all died of. I am concerned about my daughter and my granddaughter

because now I have given them a tremendous risk factor. I feel like I have, I feel like I have given the succeeding generations of women in my family a huge risk factor. Not by choice, but it bothers me that they now have this immense risk factor.

Julia feels liable, accountable. Her gene pool undergoes mutation; the bloodline alters. She opens the risk for cancer. Developing cancer carries a heavy familial burden.

Julia's Beliefs about Cancer

Estrogens and viruses are central to Julia's beliefs about cancer causation. She echoes the latest knowledge offered by science. The power of science, however, is tempered with the reality of cancer. For Julia, breast cancer is beyond science at this time in medicine's development.

I think in breast cancer, I'm reasonably convinced that it has something to do with estrogens. Because all of the risk factors that are associated with the development of the disease are tied to some point in a woman's life when her estrogen or her hormonal levels change. It has to do with the onset of menstruation, when, whether she's had children and what age she had children, so that somehow I think it's associated with, with hormones. In what way, I don't know. And I really don't think they're very close to figuring it out either. There's the whole business about oncogenes, which I really don't know a lot about, but I don't put, for example, a lot of credence in dietary causation. I understand the association between, say, a high fat diet and the potential development of breast cancer, but again that may be hormonal. The fats may cause the estrogens to be retained more because it's, it's tied with the fat or something like that.

An informed and educated woman, Julia has her own ideas about the genesis of cancer. She thinks that cancer may also be caused by a virus. "I wonder if it is some kind of a slow virus or something that we pick up, and it just takes a long time for it to do whatever it is."

I very strongly believe that it's not, that you don't cause your own cancer kind of thing. There was a lovely letter in a journal that I received by a woman who said, "You are not going to make me think I caused my cancer." I don't mean to minimize the place, the part that individuals can have in dealing with cancer. But I don't, I don't put a lot of credence in [the idea that] if you have the right thoughts, you can [laughs] you can keep your cancer from recurring, or you're gonna make it go away and all that kind of stuff. One of the big gurus in the United States [who proposes this] — I detest his body of literature. I think he really does emphasize that, if you had dealt with all the bad relationships in your life why you wouldn't have gotten cancer. And I think this lays a horrendous guilt trip on people. That's another thing that annoys me. I think he's making a mint on people who are desperate for something that reassures them.

Julia is not the cause of her cancer. A book on "positive thoughts" makes her furious. People with cancer are often desperate. They seek what science and the health care system cannot offer them. Consumed by cancer, they embark on pilgrimages searching for hope, for a cure, or at least for reassurances — only to be devoured by something else, by someone else. Desperation makes for easy prey.

Julia is also wary about alternative therapies. Some of her friends who have breast cancer make use of alternative treatments. Julia does not, in great measure, because of her life experiences.

My nursing background contributes to my scepticism of alternative treatments … they don't seem to have a real good hard scientific base yet. I know there's this whole body of literature out there that's beginning to develop about immunology and the effect of the emotions and things on immunology. I guess I'm just too sceptical to invest a great deal of time and effort. Plus I already have the disease. I don't honestly believe that there is something that I can consciously do that's going to keep it from coming back.

Scepticism prevents Julia from investing in alternative therapies. Alternative modalities are not an option for her. Julia believes that cancer is beyond her consciousness and she can do nothing that will prevent it from coming back. Chemotherapy, radiation, herbal teas, the power of positive thinking — none of these will stop Julia's cancer if it decides to come back.

Breast Cancer: Diagnosis and the Treatment

Julia detects a lump in her breast during April of 1990. Given her history of fibrocystic breast disease, she is used to the presence of lumps in her breast. This lump feels different. It is hard; she could roll it around in her fingers. Anxious about the lump and its lack of familiarity, Julia senses its danger, knows it is cancer.

I found a lump in my left breast in April of 1990. I had a history of recurrent "fibrocystic disease" and had a number of lumps aspirated and biopsied, but this one felt different. And in my mind I knew from the moment I found it that it was cancer. I went to see my family doctor and she said she wanted me to see a surgeon. And she said, "You'll be back." And I said, "What for?" And then she said, "For your pre-surgical physical." And I said, "So you think I'm going to have surgery." And the doctor said, "Yes, I think so." But she never once used the word cancer. And she never once said, "I think it's cancer, I think it's serious," or anything like that.

The family physician recognizes Julia's bodily understanding. Something heinous resides in Julia's breast, something unspeakable. Both Julia and her physician sense that the lump is cancer. Their beliefs must be validated by a higher authority — a surgeon. Julia consults the surgeon. He dismisses the possibility of cancer. From his perspective, the lump buried in her breast is symptomatic of fibrocystic breast disease.

I got in to see the surgeon later that week. He examined me and said, "I think we're dealing with the same thing we've always dealt with. I think it is just another lump." And I said, "What if it's not?" And he said, "Julia, I'm 99 percent sure that it's the same kind of lump as before. Let's do what we've always done. Go through one menstrual cycle and then biopsy it if it is still there."

Concerns are easily dismissed when they are about bodies-at-a-distance. This space between physician and patient provides cool objectivity and no emotional heat. Julia's observations are discredited. She is too close to the problem, too close to the lump in her breast. The lump, according to the surgeon, is not cancerous. This lump proves him wrong.

Waiting, at the request of the surgeon, Julia continues with her life's routine. Even though she is certain the lump will not disappear with the completion of a menstrual cycle, she does not prompt the surgeon for immediate action. Instead, she follows the surgeon's instructions. The lump remains despite the completion of her menstrual cycle. Julia has a biopsy.

I chose to have a two-step procedure. I wanted the biopsy first and I wanted
a frozen section done so I knew the results before I left the hospital. So ... it
was malignant ... [in a soft voice] ... adenocarcinoma. The physician came
out and told my husband that it was cancer. I was in the out-patient department and they took me and my husband into a cubicle. I could tell by the
look on my husband's face and I ... said, "What's the matter?" He said,
"It's cancer." And he started crying. I didn't start crying because I knew. I
just knew what it was going to be. And it didn't bother me that the surgeon
did not tell me, but it was hard for my husband to tell me. It was hard
on *him.*

Julia's lump is cancerous — adenocarcinoma. She has invasive cancer of the cells lining the milk ducts of her breast. The surgeon does not
speak directly to her. He speaks to her husband. Telling, when there is
an error in prediction, has its chain of command. Michael cries when
he tells his wife the bad news. Julia does not cry. She knew the diagnosis before she consulted the surgeon.

Julia seeks a second opinion, a second surgeon, and perhaps a
second chance. The surgeons are in agreement about the diagnosis and
the treatment. A mastectomy is required.

I got a second opinion from another surgeon. She said that with surgery and
adequate treatment that I would have between an 80 percent to 90 percent
chance of a five year survival time. The odds that the first surgeon gave me
were about 75 percent. I came back and I scheduled the mastectomy. It
was very important to me to know what all my choices were and for me to
pick out what I wanted, how I wanted to do it, and when I wanted the
mastectomy.

Julia now knows the odds of surviving her breast cancer. Having
this information is important since she actively engages in making decisions about her disease. She wants as much information as possible.
There are things that she can do to improve her chances of survival:
gathering information and making her own decisions. Julia does not
permit cancer to erode her independence, who she is as a person.

Julia weathers the mastectomy and does well in surgery. She is elat-
ed when she hears that she is "node negative" and that her bone scan is
clear. Cancer is limited to her breast. It is not present in the lymph
nodes under her arm. Julia is relieved that the cancer is contained.
Her emotions are similarly contained at this point. Yet, the details of

daily living move her to tears. She is compelled to reflect upon her circumstances.

> I got ready for bed and I couldn't get my nightgown on because I couldn't raise my arm. And then I started crying. It was probably the first time I cried … I cried … I started crying and my husband said, "Of all the things we've been through and this makes you cry? A nightgown is going to cause us problems?" Eventually, I got into the nightgown.

What is tolerable during the day cannot be endured at night. Julia cannot slip on her nightgown. Unable to dress herself for bed, she dissolves into tears. Julia finally acknowledges what she has been through, what has happened to her body, to herself, to her life. She cries in recognition of her ordeal. Sympathy for the self, at last.

Julia rallies. Within two weeks of her surgery she decides to go swimming. She does not permit the cancer to completely dominate her life.

> I asked my doctor if it was okay to go swimming. He said it was okay. So I went swimming two weeks after I had surgery. I swam a quarter of a mile, not a very graceful stroke or anything. But I was swimming. It was kind of a strange-looking sidestroke, but I could swim.

Julia takes to the freedom of water. Wounded, she swims with a distinct lack of grace. Swimming soothes her; she embraces life.

Taking Chemotherapy and Making Choices

In July 1990 Julia commences chemotherapy. She opts not to take adriamycin, which from Julia's perspective is the strongest of all cancer medications. As a witness to the plight of other women, Julia knows about the possible side effects of this drug.

> I got methotrexate, 5FU and cytoxin. Treatment for breast cancer is probably one of the most standardized treatments for cancer that there is, and so when I talk about making choices, in some ways I didn't have a choice. The physician recommended adriamycin over methotrexate, but I knew from experience, I knew what adriamycin could do. I mean I know how much people threw up and that you automatically lost your hair. I didn't want to deal with adria, so I said, "No, I'd rather have methotrexate." So I started

chemotherapy. I was premenopausal throughout this and I started my period
the day I started my chemo. [loudly, with excitement in her voice] And it
was wonderful! I thought, "My God, my body can do something normal."
Because my body was just doing so many awful things. That was the last
period I had up to today.

Julia refuses to take "adria." The day she commences chemotherapy, she starts her period. She welcomes her menstruation and the
reassurance that her body has not completely betrayed her. "My God,
my body can do something normal." Something normal, something
not malignant. Despite her attempts to control the side effects of
chemotherapy, Julia experiences difficulties.

I started losing my hair and I was nauseated. I was constantly nauseated, but
I never did throw up. I had some diarrhea — that was really uncomfortable.
I was really tired and my bone marrow got depressed [chemotherapy can
reduce the production of blood cells by the bone marrow]. In September,
my foot began to hurt, but I kind of ignored it. I got a book from the library
and it said that methotrexate sometimes causes bone pain. So I went in and
told my doctor about it. He said not to worry about it. By the following
week, it really hurt. I returned to the clinic and said, "I think I've got blood
clots." And the nurse checked me. The nurse called the oncologist and he
was annoyed. So the nurse then called my family physician and she said,
"Well, we better do a venogram" [to see if there were blood clots in the veins
of her leg]. The venogram was positive and I had blood clots. They admitted me straight away into the hospital. I ended up spending a week in the
hospital, in bed.

Hair loss, nausea, diarrhea, bone marrow depression, and blood
clots. Body losses; the purge of chemotherapy. As a nurse, Julia knows
something is terribly wrong. This is the second time in her cancer experience when her knowledge of the intricate workings and feelings of her
body are not acknowledged. Her concerns seem to be an annoyance to
the oncologist. There are risks in having an opinion and questioning
medical authorities. Once tests reveal the scientific truth and legitimize
her personal knowledge, Julia is admitted to the hospital.

Julia asserts herself. Decision making around her cancer treatment
is a means to an end. Control, not of cancer but of the consequences of
its treatment. Making decisions about her treatment is self-empower-
ing, it is a matter of self-preservation. It is a matter of survival.

I wanted some testing done on my tumour which the doctors do not routinely do here. I wanted flow cytometric measurements of S-phase and ploidy [a test to determine the growth capacity of the tumour; its ability to reproduce], and the reason I wanted it done was that I had read some stuff that said that it's a good prognostic indicator of recurrence. And the physician's philosophy was that it wouldn't change what they would do for me. I said, "No, but it may change what I want to do, and it may also change what kind of decisions I make about my life." If the prognostic indicators came back that I was really susceptible or really vulnerable to recurrence, then I'm going to set some different priorities and make some different choices about how I'm going to conduct my life.

The specific tests that Julia requests will indicate her susceptibility to cancer recurrence. The physician, looking "at" Julia rather than looking "with" her, notes that her treatment modality will not change regardless of the test results. Persistent in her efforts to have these tests, Julia attempts to have her physicians hear her life beyond her cancer cells. From the other side, from the receiving end of things, from Julia's perspective, the chromocytometry results matter. Julia may make different choices about her life. Priorities might be reordered. Her physician orders these special tests. They reveal that Julia's cancer is likely to recur.

Cytometric measurements show how much of the tumour is in the "S" phase, which is the bad phase for the tumour to be in. There's aneuploid, diploid ... anyway, I had an aneuploid tumour and that's not good. And I had a high "S" phase which isn't good either. And so that was important to me to know.

The chance of recurrence is high since Julia's tumour is in a bad phase. Julia now knows that her cancer may seed and take root beyond her breast. Her concerns change. She speaks of the odds of dying. Julia makes the connection between cancer and death. "I know what my odds are and my odds stink." The odds favour Julia's cancer.

Waiting out Cancer: The First Scare

The physicians monitor Julia's body at three month intervals. X-rays, blood tests, and palpation of her chest are conducted to rule out the advance of cancer. Life is lived from check-up to check-up. The potential for bad news looms. Julia experiences anxiety, angst, and uncertainty a week or so before each of her check-ups. Tension develops both in her body and in her mind. Tension builds until the outcome of her tests for that interval are known.

I got half-way through in 1992 and went in for, I was still going in for a check-up every three months. It got, it had just been extended out to four months for my check-up and I was to go in on a Thursday in June of last year. I always wondered in my mind, what am I, what, how am I going to react and what is the doctor going to say if the cancer comes back. What is the doctor going to say if it comes back? One time during that year he walked in with an X-ray beside him and he said, "Julia, I want you to look at this." And I thought, "Oh shit!" And yet I just took it fairly calmly. And he popped the X-ray on the viewer and there was a spot up there and he said, "I want to do a lung scan." And I said, "No! That's been there before. If you look at the other X-rays you'll see it." And he said, "We don't have any other X-rays." And I said, "I'll get you some." So I insisted that they get my X-rays from this other clinic. He got the other X-rays and that spot had been there for years. That was the first scare.

Julia is her own patient advocate. Knowledge is power and Julia knows things. She knows about her body and cancer. The spot of this X-ray is not indicative of a cancer march. Julia instructs her physician to compare this X-ray with previous X-rays. He does and she is right. Julia is about to live out her fear of recurrence.

Waiting out Cancer: Recurrence

The cytometric measurements prove prophetic. Julia's cancer spreads. Despite the chemotherapy and the constant monitoring, it seeds.

I went in for my check-up in June 1992. The doctor did an exam and was checking over my scar and he said, "Put your arm up here." And he felt down the mastectomy scar and he found a lump under the scar. He said, "There's a lump here." And I said, "Really?" Because I was, I wasn't great about checking it and I hadn't felt it. It was a tumour hidden between two muscles. The only time you felt it was when your arm was back and the muscle slid out. And I hadn't checked the scar in that position.

A covert swelling is discovered under Julia's scar line. Hidden, it thrives undetected between two muscles, beyond the reach of Julia's searching fingers. The lump is removed in the oncologist's office. An ancient ceremony repeats itself. Julia's flesh is read; a portend for the future. Her flesh does not bode well for her.

Michael and I were sitting on the porch and I said, "My cancer's back." And Michael said, "How do you know?" And then I told him about the tumour. And that was a turning point because he told me, he said, "You know, when you were first diagnosed and they gave you the odds of 75 percent chance of a five-year survival, I figured we had a fighting chance and that things would be okay." My odds are now one-in-four, not much, a 25 percent chance of surviving the next five years. Michael said, "When your odds drop that much, I don't trust the cancer." So his trust and optimism about my long-term survival is not good.

Julia's chances of surviving the next five years are greatly reduced with the discovery of the lump along her mastectomy scar. Her husband no longer trusts the cancer. He is less optimistic. He becomes concerned. Julia's doctors initiate a battery of tests and the number and type of tests reflect the seriousness of her situation. She requires a metastatic work-up.

You have to go through a metastatic work-up to see if the cancer is anyplace else. They did a bone scan and they did a CT scan of the liver — and I had some spots on my liver which scared me — I told myself I am not ready for cancer to be in my liver. I can deal, I think I can deal with it being in my chest and being a local recurrence, but I kept thinking I'm not ready for it to be metastasized. They had to do a liver biopsy because they didn't know for sure what the spots were and they had to find out. I had a liver biopsy done and it was normal. The spots were just cysts. The chest X-ray was okay and the blood indicators of whether the cancer had returned were also okay.

Cancer on the move has its favourite hiding places: the liver, the lung, bones. Secret flesh within flesh. Julia's oncologists pry into her body core. CT scans, X-rays, and blood work confirm a localized recurrence. Although her odds are now greatly reduced, Julia still has a chance of surviving her cancer.

The physicians recommend a six-month cycle of chemotherapy. Julia obtains a second opinion. There is consensus. She must undergo another round of chemotherapy. In preparation for the treatments, Julia requests a medication port.

I had a port [A device placed under the skin and sewn into a vein near the collarbone. It permits repeated administration of medications and chemotherapy without having to start an IV each time] put in, in advance of the treatment. And they put it in an awful place. I was in a considerable amount of pain for a week and I, I told my physician that this was not working. I said, "It has got to come out. You've got to put it some place else. I can't stand this." So I had that first port taken out and another one put in. I said, "Don't you ever put one of those things in somebody there again!"

Port, from the Latin "portus" meaning harbour, a place of refuge. For the physicians, it is the route to Julia's cancer; the entrance to a body under siege. It will protect Julia's veins from being burned by the chemotherapy. Julia also receives concurrent radiation treatments. "I took radiation for six weeks, finished it in early September." Her cancer is aggressive. It seeded during her initial chemotherapy treatments. Controlling the cancer now requires a combination of chemotherapy and radiation.

Living with Breast Cancer: A Path of Uncertainty

Julia's life revolves around check-ups. A constant, patterned monitoring of her body takes place. Every three months Julia must face the fact that she is a person with cancer and that her cancer may be advancing. It is a forced encounter with the possibility of mortality.

The doctor had me coming in every three months for a check-up. They always do blood work, which is a CBC [complete blood count] and a chemistry pattern. Every other visit they do a chest X-ray. I was due to come back in June 1993 and I was having some back pain which scared me and I told my physician about it during my last visit. He said, "Well, we probably ought to be doing a bone scan." Because I've already had a recurrence, I suspect they'll do bone scans every year. Last Friday I had a bone scan done, and all the blood work, a chest X-ray and a mammogram. And I was really scared about the bone scan because I've been having back pain. And so I debated. Do I want to call and get the results before the long weekend? Or do I want to wait because my appointment to go in and see the doctor is tomorrow. I called. And everything was fine and I was delighted. The nurse said, "It's fine, other than you've got arthritis in your knees."

Minor body ailments, aches and pains, cannot be ignored. Their presence can herald migration. The source of Julia's back pain may be cancer, her bones protesting the presence of an intruder. But the pain is a simple ache of some kind. Julia is delighted and she can momentarily stop wondering, "What if it is back?" Despite the reassurances, there are no guarantees that cancer will not surface. That profound trust between the self and the body is forever breached. The spectre of another recurrence is always present.

I had about worked myself to the point, between my original diagnosis and when I found out, when the recurrence was found … I had just started to kind of relax and think, "Okay, maybe this disease is not going to come back and I'm going to be okay" … and then it came back. I just can't completely trust that the disease is not going to rear its ugly head again. I don't know how long it will be before I can be completely relaxed about it. For right now I'm willing to think, "Okay, things are going alright. They've done all their 'big tests' that can be done. If they can't find anything there, then there's nothing there."

The "big tests" — bone scans, CT scans, and biopsies — do not reveal cancer. "If they can't find anything there, then there's nothing there." Negative results offer Julia a chance to catch her breath, to enjoy a reprieve from cancer, no matter how transitory.

It's a liberating kind of thing that once you, you kind of know, okay, at this point, it's not there. You can kind of start again to push it back or not let it occupy so much of your thoughts. And you can be a little bit freer about planning.

Living with breast cancer entails an ebb and flow of uncertainty. There is knowing and then not knowing whether cancer has advanced any further. Cancer moves in cycles: anxiety, check-ups, and relief. Julia discovers that each phase has a rhythm. She learns the cadences associated with cancer — the measures, the waiting, and the fear. Living with cancer is a life of uncertainty.

Although her cancer is in abeyance, if it mobilizes, nothing will likely be able to stop it. It is as if Julia's cancer has its own agenda, a will. Julia is certain of this.

A friend of mine asked me one time, she said, "Julia, do you really think that you can keep your cancer from coming back?" And I said, "No. If it's going to come back, it's going to come back." Some people may think this is fatalistic and when I talk with friends about the statistics that I face, they suggest that maybe I'll be in the 25 percent who make it. I don't know. I don't really think there's any way that I can necessarily do anything particular that's going to make me be in that 25 percent as opposed to the 75 percent of people who experience another recurrence.

Julia thinks she may be perceived as fatalistic. She will fall, however, into one statistical group or the other: remission or recurrence. According to Julia, such things often happen by chance. She knows that at present the chances of recurrence are greater. She may be more realistic than pessimistic. "I can't do anything. I just have to learn to live with the fact that the disease may come back and if it comes back it may kill me." Julia cannot do anything. Since her cancer may return, may come out of hiding and kill her, Julia believes it is necessary to consider this reality. Cancer is a hard cold truth. For Julia, acknowledging cancer's death threat makes living possible. The possibility of her death becomes a part of living for both Julia and her husband.

Julia observes that people die of cancer. Photographs of cancer survivors claim, "Cancer Can Be Beaten." They are proof of progress in the treatment of this disease. Julia, however, is more familiar with the cancer deaths. The names of the dead and their pictures are not circulated. Claimed by cancer, they are hidden from view, buried in the back pages of newspapers. Obituaries announce their encounters with cancer, their struggles, and their eventual deaths. Some are described as valiant and courageous and having fought a battle.

There are some cancers that appear to respond well to treatment. But to me, it's not the majority of them. The more I've read this stuff … there's all these, quote, "survivors" out there, but I don't know where they are. The people I know … most of us have had recurrences and some of us are dying. There's a couple of women in the support group who were diagnosed seven or eight years ago. They're doing fine. And maybe the people who are doing fine don't ever come out to the support group meetings and they get on with their lives. And you don't know they had cancer, but I don't know that it's a beatable disease. I know more people who have died of cancer than I know who have survived.

The people Julia knows have suffered recurrences. And, "Some of us are dying." Julia includes herself among the dying. Five years is the golden standard. If you are not dead by the end of that time, the story goes, you have managed to beat cancer. But cancer does not respect time frames, and people are dying of cancer beyond the five years. "Once it comes back, your chances of long-term survival are just about zip." The slogan, "Cancer Can Be Beaten," demoralizes Julia. It minimizes her plight. It casts her as a failure.

I think those kinds of things, "Cancer Can Be Beaten," make it difficult for those of us who have had cancer because it minimizes what we're dealing with. People, when you say something to them, they will give you a variety of survival stories. Oh, I know so-and-so, aunt, uncle, who had such-and-such cancer and they are doing fine and that was 20 years ago. That's one version you get. The other one is, "Oh, they're doing so much research and there's so many new, new things coming. I know you'll just be fine." Those are the two most common kind of public reactions. And so then that kind of leaves those of us that have had cancer, it makes it easier for people to dismiss us. Oh, you are going to be okay because "cancer can be beaten."

Cancer Treatment: A Crap Shoot

Julia's faith in her check-ups begins to wane. Her optimism fades. Her perspective becomes negative. According to Julia, successful treatment of breast cancer is unpredictable.

Basically it's a crap shoot. There is a fairly standard treatment and the oncologists give it to you and if it works — that's great. But they have no idea whether it's going to work or not. Now I got to thinking after I went in for my check-up last week. Why do I even go in? Because the whole idea of going in for check-ups is predicated on the fact that the physicians will catch it early if it comes back. So what are they going to do if it comes back? If it comes back, that means that I have failed every standard treatment that there is. There isn't anything left to do except maybe give me medications that I've taken before or maybe give me some radiation. But there isn't anything else that the oncologists can really do for me if the cancer comes back. So why do I go in and have all this stuff done? So what if they find it … what are they going to do?

At one time, Julia's visits to her oncologists were for security, for reassurance that her cancer had not spread. This sense of security transforms into pessimism. Julia becomes a cancer cynic. Detecting the early spread of cancer is now meaningless to her situation. She has already experienced a local recurrence — a metastasis, a new tumour along her scar line. Further metastases, beyond the geography of her scar line, would dramatically change the course of her cancer path. Another recurrence means that she has failed every standard treatment for breast cancer.

Cancer in a temporary state of quiet means living on the edge of life. And on the edge of death. Julia is acutely aware of the false securities offered by the blood tests, X-rays, CT scans, and other measures. In a period of three months, a person's fate can change dramatically.

The Terror of Cancer Dreams

Julia has cancer dreams. Cancer invades her psyche, to the very depths of her being. Night terrors. Julia speaks of pure fear.

Some time within the last month I woke up screaming one night. Michael shook me and I know he was saying, "Julia, Julia, Julia, wake up!" And I was in the throes of some kind of dream. That was the scariest dream I've had. I was terrified and I was in some kind of situation where I was very, very threatened. I don't remember the details other than being terrified. Feeling very threatened and trying to grasp hold of something to help me or save me or something. And the scary part of it is that, I think that my body is trying to tell me something. Am I dying? And I don't know it yet. My body telling my mind something that isn't physically obvious yet.

Terrorized by a malignant threat, Julia tries to grasp hold of something to help her, to save her. The dream frightens Julia and the message within the dream invokes dread. Her body is aware of imminent danger. The horror of this dream comes to light, softened now in the daytime telling. Her body leads Julia to ask, "Am I dying?" Julia wakes up screaming at her predicament, at the possibility that cancer is advancing undetected in her body.

Cancer as Metaphor: A Touchstone

Julia describes her cancer as a touchstone — a fine-grained stone used to test the value of gold and silver by the colour of the streak made on it — over which she draws her life. "With this touchstone, it's almost been a solidification of who I am." Cancer, a hard, cold, stone, enables Julia to appreciate the value of her life, her accomplishments, and the dreams she has realized.

I finally decided that for me, cancer is a touchstone. Touchstone. It's like a point that allows you to identify the values and things that are important to you. I guess a touchstone originally was a black stone that merchants would scratch gold across to see, to decide on the value of the gold or the silver, to determine the value of the bullion. I think touchstone describes it best because I have pulled my life across cancer and decided what's valuable to me.

In addition to the terrible things that cancer brings, it also presents opportunities for reflection. An inward journey. Cancer affords Julia the chance to review her life, to take comfort in those things that are meaningful to her.

With cancer we've been given a chance that most people or a lot of people don't get. We're faced with a life-threatening disease and have the opportunity to re-evaluate our lives. And I don't think that most people sit down and evaluate their lives as to what's meaningful and do something about it.

Cancer provides Julia with a chance to change her life. She alters her priorities. Relationships with family members and friends now take precedence in her life. Relationships matter.

I think the relationships in my life are much more important to me now than a whole lot more of the other stuff. You know, I still do my work and I think I do a good job with it, but the relationships in my life are more important.

Thoughts on Dying

Julia begins to speak of dying and death. One day at the swimming pool, she sobs uncontrollably in the shower. How would she tell her grandchild, Louise, that she was dying? Thoughts of death surface more and more as Julia's journey speeds up and she moves further away from the land of the well.

I know who will write my obituary. In fact, he will probably write it before I die. And I do not want it to say that I was a victim of cancer, or that I died after a long battle. I don't want military metaphors and victimization. I would rather it said something like, "She faced cancer with grace." I haven't written my obituary, but I know what I don't want said. I don't know what I'll be like if cancer comes back and what I actually will feel like in the dying process.

I don't know what I'll be like. I might be an absolute old bitch [laughter] and so maybe I won't die with grace. So far, I've tried to be graceful.

Throughout her cancer journey, Julia tries to be a good cancer patient, a good wife, mother, and grandmother. She manages as best she can. Julia wants to face death with grace, but cancer may rob her of this and make her an "absolute old bitch" who dies without grace.

Julia continually mentions the possibility that her cancer may return. She wrestles with the thought of resuming chemotherapy. "I don't know if I could go through with chemo again." Choices around cancer are never easy.

If it comes back again it's probably going to kill me regardless of what the physicians do. I think I'd rather go ahead and cram whatever things I really wanted to do into the time I had left before I started to feel the effects of the return of cancer. If I took chemo, I wouldn't feel good again until I died.

Julia feels vulnerable. If her cancer metastasizes, Julia may seize what is left of her life and enjoy those moments free of the effects of chemotherapy. "If the doctors have their way, they will just keep you on chemotherapy until you die. You'd just be going through hell before you die." Again.

During a check-up in March 1994, Julia's oncologist informs her that her cancer has spread to her lungs and bones. Her worst nightmare is realized. Julia cannot now awaken from the terrors of the darkest hours of the night.

I've been home sick for a couple of days. I now have bilateral pleural effusions [fluid on both her lungs] and I am going into the hospital to have one drained on Friday. I also have bronchitis and I am coughing a lot. The unknown continues to be scary. The effusions are due to the cancer. I did not expect it to progress so rapidly. I thought I would have more time to ease into dying. The suddenness of the new symptoms brings forth the desire to want to grasp at chemo or something to slow down the cancer so that I can adjust.

*

Julia refuses to take a final round of chemotherapy. In the fall of 1994 she died — with grace.

*

I see it [the divine] in the laughs and smiles of my grandchildren, in the geese as they begin their flight south, in Michael as he walked ahead of me down a path in the forests of Australia. I even see it in Dad when he enjoys a walk outside with me. These are the blessings that having cancer gives me — the opportunity to see the world in a way that I think many people miss because they have not been threatened with the loss of all that is meaningful to them. Even if I do lose it all through death, I will treasure the view that I have had.

— Julia, October 5, 1993

LESSONS LEARNED: JULIA'S GIFTS TO US

Julia invited us to accompany her on the breast cancer path. Although we may feel saddened about her suffering — and the tragedy of her death — Julia wanted her story shared with women and other cancer patients. Helpful, always, to women with breast cancer, Julia believed that sharing the details of her experience would benefit women, their partners, family members, and others in their lives. Knowing what happened to Julia helps us comprehend what can be encountered on the breast cancer path. Artists portray fearful things in life — dehumanization, suffering, and death — not for shock value, but to capture an understanding of the worst possible things and thereby tame them. Paint, bronze, marble, and words give shape to our suffering. We "see" and experience for ourselves, from a safe distance, the objects of our terror. What becomes familiar or understood is often less feared. And so Julia offers us gifts through her account of dying from breast cancer.

Engaging in Life

Julia seized every minute of every day while living with breast cancer. She did not take life and love for granted. Living with cancer was difficult, however, and Julia made a conscious decision to try not to let cancer completely dominate her life. She swam, she went birding with her husband, she babysat her grandchildren, and took time to offer support to other women with breast cancer. She sought out the company of her good friends. This was not simply hiding in the hurly-burly of life. Julia did what was important to her as a person living with the uncertainty of cancer, enjoying the company of those she loved and those who loved her. Julia also ensured quiet moments in her life.

Solitude and the need to reflect upon her life were also important to Julia. She took time out for herself, her needs, her interests. Julia wrote her thoughts with the intention of writing a book about her experiences. Although initially faithful to this task, she abandoned this project once her cancer advanced and her energy diminished.

- ◆ Whenever possible, continue those activities in life that are rewarding and which provide solace. Who we are is often found in what we do. Remaining engaged in life and living as fully as possible is important.

- ◆ Many cancer hardships are surmountable through love. Surround yourself with loving family and friends.

- ◆ Keeping life as normal as possible provides people with the comfort found in familiar things and routines. This does not imply that you have to be a "superman" or a "superwoman" and "do it all" while living with cancer. You may temporarily stop some of your routines (because of treatment side effects and symptoms), however, many routines can be maintained through careful pacing and planning.

- ◆ Do what is possible given how you feel and how much energy you have at your disposal. When you feel sick or exhausted, don't do anything. Rest. Take the phone off the hook. Have a friend babysit children for the afternoon. Take some time for yourself when you are feeling bad.

- ◆ Cancer can isolate us from life and those who love us. Reach out to family and friends. Let them know what they can do to be of help and of comfort. Often people do not know what to say or what to do when they learn that someone they care for has cancer. They may "shy away" from you. You may need to take the initiative to stay connected with certain family members and friends.

Cancer competes with our lives. It can isolate us from our bodies, our family, and friends. It takes us from the land of the well into a world of sickness where disfigurement, nausea, vomiting, diminishing energy, pain, and suffering become part of our living. Julia knew this happened to people with cancer and so she actively engaged in life. It was Julia's decision to not permit cancer to isolate her from living as fully as possible.

Living in the Present and for the Future

Julia did not assume that there would be a tomorrow; cancer robs us of the certainty of tomorrow. Each day was remarkable and held wonder for her. Julia paused, took stock of her life, and realized what she had — a loving spouse, good children, cherished grandchildren, and caring friends and colleagues. Her life and struggle with cancer mattered to others. She knew she was loved and she loved others. Relationships with special people in her life became a priority. Julia let go of some relationships; the ones that were not nurturing or authentic.

- Take stock of what is important to you. Reinforce, nurture, and protect those things in your life that are meaningful, validating, and sustaining.

- When you can, let go of those things that cause you stress, discomfort, or drain your energy. If you can't let go, figure out how things can be less taxing to you.

- Think of yourself. Be kind to yourself. Take care of yourself.

- Don't be afraid to show sympathy-for-the-self. This is not wallowing in self-pity. It is recognizing that something terrible is happening to you. Acknowledging and understanding what has happened to you is an important part of healing. Tears can be cathartic and they may be helpful for inner healing.

- Change those things that need to be and can be changed. Although difficult, try to accept those things in your life that cannot be changed.

Acknowledging cancer's death threat made Julia more fully alive — something that comes too late for many of us. Cancer offered Julia a chance to change things in her life before she died.

Participating in Your Cancer Care

It was important to Julia to be active in her cancer care. But becoming knowledgeable about cancer and wanting a say in its treatment also has its risks. Not all physicians are comfortable with people who know enough to challenge them on decisions or who express a desire to participate in making decisions.

- If you want to take an active role in your cancer experience, you need to communicate this wish to your physician. Let your physician know right from the start — your first encounter with him or her — that you want to make informed choices concerning your cancer treatment.

- Considerable information about cancer is available to you from many sources: health care providers, the Cancer Society, on the Internet, at your local public library or university library, and from friends and family members. Support groups also offer members information about cancer. You need to be informed if you want to participate in decision making about living with cancer.

- If you want an active role in your cancer care and your physician is not willing to work with you, then find another physician who will. It is important to feel that you and your physician are supportive and respectful of each other.

- Ask about treatment options. Find out what treatment choices are available to you as a person who is living with cancer.

Julia recognized that indicating her choices was accompanied by risks, but she chose an active role nonetheless. For example, she requested a two-step procedure to first confirm the presence of cancer in her breast and then to treat it. In a two-step procedure, the diagnosis of breast cancer is made first by a pathologist examining a sample of breast tissue under a microscope, and then surgery is done on another day. These two steps provide surgeons and women with cancer some time to consider treatment options. The time between confirmation of the diagnosis and surgery permitted Julia to prepare herself physically and emotionally for what was to happen to her.

People living with cancer are often encouraged to be positive and hopeful throughout their experience. Julia was realistic, although some of her friends and caregivers interpreted her stance as pessimistic. She was courageous in that she sought the truth about her cancer, about the odds of surviving her disease. This was Julia's way. She wanted to know what her chances were so that she could make decisions about her life and her dying. Julia was hopeful and positive about surviving, but she did not operate under false pretences. Although this knowledge can be frightening, it enabled Julia to make plans, to live out her life the best she could given the reality of her circumstances.

Obtaining a Second Opinion

When Julia was initially informed of her cancer she sought the opinion of a second surgeon. This was in keeping with Julia's desire to obtain information about her cancer and to have a "say" in what happened to her as a person with cancer.

- Second opinions are not a waste of time or money. If you want a second opinion — get one! Not only is it your right as a person living with cancer, a second opinion can provide you with peace of mind.

- Ask your physician to recommend and refer you for a second opinion. Your physician will be able to forward information to this second physician.

- Don't feel guilty about asking for a second opinion. This is your life and your cancer experience. You need to believe that your treatment is appropriate and necessary.

Julia wanted to present her situation, and the lump in her breast, to another surgeon. The second surgeon confirmed the diagnosis and proposed treatment plan. A mastectomy was required. Assured that a mastectomy was important and necessary, Julia consented to this procedure.

The Need for Talking and Emotional Support

Julia experienced terrible nightmares. She feared a recurrence of cancer and felt that her body was speaking to her through her dreams. She also experienced periods of intense anxiety when she was due for a check-up which could herald the recurrence of cancer. Living with cancer was fraught with uncertainty, fear, and terror. She eventually came to terms with this anxiety when she recognized that she could not control her cancer.

- Nightmares are terrifying. Should you repeatedly experience nightmares, you may want to consider talking with someone, formally or informally, to help you come to terms with the terror in your dreams.

- Anxiety and fear are often experienced by people living with cancer prior to "cancer check-ups." If this happens to you, talking with someone may help you work through and manage these feelings. Cancer is frightening and you do not have to "hang tough" with your fears and anxieties. If you do not wish to go for counselling or cannot afford it, identify someone that you can talk to in confidence about your fears.

- Some people find that support groups help them as they live with cancer. Fellow cancer journeyers understand what is happening to you — because it is happening to them. Support groups offer their members mutual support and caring.

Julia tended to deal with her fear and anxiety on her own. Although she facilitated some support groups, she did not seek help regarding her own fears. In retrospect, Julia might have benefited from talking to a counsellor, her physician, her oncology nurse, or someone who could have assisted her in understanding and managing these fears.

Finding Your Voice in the Cancer Experience

There were occasions when Julia had to demand that her physicians listen to her. She observed changes in her body, and when she tried to tell the physicians and nurses about these things, her concerns were dismissed, ignored, or trivialized. Julia knew something was wrong with her foot. She developed pain in her foot while she was taking chemotherapy and she was aware of the side effects associated with that particular chemotherapeutic medication. Julia informed her physician about this symptom. "He said not to worry about it." The pain did not ease and Julia returned to the clinic where she was able to mobilize a nurse to contact another physician about her problem. When her family physician eventually ordered a test, it confirmed that Julia had developed blood clots in the veins of her foot. She was then admitted to a hospital for treatment.

Sometimes our voices are not viewed as legitimate by the health care community — they are subjective, emotional, lack factual foundation, and can easily be dismissed. In contrast, our bodies are heard through technology: X-rays, CT scans, blood tests. These are the things that speak to many of the members of the medical community. Having cancer, however, sometimes requires us to speak out and rage against being silenced.

- ◆ Women's observations about their bodies may be dismissed or trivialized by some members of the medical establishment. If you think that something is wrong with your body, and your physician does not seem receptive, then find another physician who will listen to you. It could save your life.

- ◆ You know your body better than anyone else. Act upon your bodily intuition. Speak out until someone listens to you.

- ◆ If you cannot find your voice, take along a close and trusted friend or family member to the physician's office who will speak for you and with you.

Julia spoke up. She spoke until someone heard her. Her voice spared her from having to undergo additional diagnostic tests and obtained necessary treatment for her blood clot. Julia communicated her choices regarding chemotherapy. She did not want to receive chemotherapy unto death. Julia had the confidence, ability, and courage to speak up. Using our voices is not always easy. Sometimes we are too frightened, or shy, or in too much pain to speak out and to raise our voices. A family member or a close friend can become our voice or can speak along with us, making a chorus commanding to be heard. Your voice can save your life. Your voice can ease the burden of your suffering. Use it.

Voicing Your Concerns as a Person Living with Cancer

Julia felt demoralized by the slogan, "Cancer Can Be Beaten." Eventually it became evident to her that she would not beat her breast cancer. By not being able to "beat cancer," Julia felt she was a failure. The message contained in this slogan suggests that perhaps she should have fought harder, or longer, or better. It also implies that Julia was somehow responsible for not responding to her treatments. The best medical practitioners and researchers have been trying to "beat" cancer and take control for over 40 years with limited success.

- If something related to your treatment, or in your experience as a person living with cancer, hurts your feelings — let people know. You are probably not the only person who is upset by slogans, treatment policies, or encounters in the clinical setting.

- Write a letter, make a phone call, send an e-mail or fax — but let people know what offends or hurts you as a person living with cancer. Your voice can prevent others from being hurt in the same way and your actions may result in people receiving better treatment.

- Talk with people who are interested and concerned about how you are being treated as a person. Agencies and clinics want to maintain good public relations and they want to offer high standards of care. Let them know what they are doing right and wrong.

- Your opinion matters. Your voice matters. You can make a difference in the lives of other people who are living with cancer.

If as a person with cancer — or as a relative or friend of someone living with cancer — you find something disturbing, then voice your concerns to the appropriate organizations. By taking action, you may not only feel better, but you may spare other people from being hurt in the same manner.

Learn How to Conduct a Breast Self-exam

Julia tried to examine her scar line and her other breast on a regular basis. She checked for new lumps. She engaged in a particular pattern when she searched for lumps. The lump under her scar line was finally detected when Julia raised her arms over her head. She had never raised her arms while conducting her breast self-exam. Probing lightly as well as deeply, lying down as well as sitting up, probing with the arm raised and then lowered may have helped Julia find this lump sooner.

- Learn how to conduct a breast self-exam (BSE).

- Encourage other women in your life (grandmothers, mothers, sisters, daughters, aunts, and nieces) to find out how to perform BSE. Then encourage them to do BSE regularly.

- Once you know how to do a BSE, make sure you conduct it on a regular basis. Make BSE a habit.

Lumps, both cancerous and benign, are often detected by women or their partners. Find out how to conduct a breast self-exam. It could save your life.

Living with Advanced Cancer

Julia wanted to die with dignity and grace. She feared cancer would rob her of this and make her a real "bitch." Julia, through her decision making and her knowledge about cancer, ensured that she died with dignity. Toward the end of her experience, she realized that cancer would claim her life. She decided not to take chemotherapy unto death. She wanted what time she had left not to be dominated by the side effects of chemotherapy. And thus, Julia took her own steps to ensure that she died with dignity.

- There may come a time when the active treatment of cancer is no longer effective.

- Palliative care — managing the symptoms of advanced cancer and ensuring comfort — can offer dignified living and dying. From a psychological perspective, letting go of active treatment can be a frightening, very difficult decision. It is a tangible admission that your cancer cannot be stopped and that you will not survive. For many people, this means giving up hope and the will to live. For others, it means acceptance and integrating dying into one's life.

- Talking with your physician and nurses about palliative care requires courage, but it can ease your suffering in the latter stages of terminal cancer. Sometimes our fear or denial of death prevents us from recognizing that death may be an inevitable part of our cancer experience.

- Palliative care is not just for the dying. It is for the living. Palliative care can help you live fully with advanced cancer.

Deciding not to continue with chemotherapy was not easy for Julia. When cancer caused changes in her ability to breathe, as it spread to her lungs, she thought about taking chemotherapy. She thought about grasping at anything that might "buy" her more time. Instead, she decided that she had received enough chemotherapy, stopped all active treatments, and instructed her doctors to keep her comfortable during the last several weeks of her life.

Julia helped us to understand the importance of engaging in life while living with cancer. Part of this process entailed pausing and "taking stock" of life. It was through reflection that Julia recognized the many sources of love in her life: her spouse, children, grandchildren, and caring friends and colleagues. Julia also showed us that being an active participant in the cancer experience was possible, but often required courage, persistence, and finding one's voice.

5

SARAH

RUNNING THE DISTANCE:
BREAST CANCER

SARAH IS A DYNAMIC WOMAN whose passion for life is remarkable. Other people are drawn to her. Articulate, a gifted listener, and well informed, Sarah's opinions matter to her family and friends. She has a wonderful sense of humour and invites laughter where ever she goes. Having lived together for eight years, Sarah and Andrew plan to marry in September. The wedding will be a celebration of their relationship, a public affirmation of their love. Sarah refers to Andrew as her soul mate. After a life of hardship, tragedy, and relationship crises, Sarah has finally found love and happiness. She considers herself fortunate to have discovered such joy at this point in her life. Andrew and Sarah live in a Victorian-era home. Their cats, Humpty and Dumpty, bring Sarah much pleasure. Like Sarah they are fiercely independent spirits.

A serious runner, Sarah displays physical stamina and fortitude. She looks younger than her 38 years. She is lean, well muscled, and toned. Sarah wears baseball caps to hide her hair loss, a recent consequence of chemotherapy. Like "the wall" in a marathon, cancer is an obstacle on Sarah's life path. It does not thwart Sarah's enthusiasm for living. She is determined to survive this disease, to run the distance. It is her ultimate race. Early in her cancer experience Sarah thinks she may be able to "outrun" the cancer. She soon realizes that cancer runs its own course. Its propensity to multiply, its tenacity and persistence to occupy Sarah's body, lead her to understand that she cannot leave cancer behind as she moves forward in life. She must run with the cancer and not away from it. Sarah cannot outdistance this disease.

Sarah's story is about a young woman whose love of life and recent happiness are assaulted by a disease. It is a tragic story of the power of cancer. This power is not absolute in that Sarah's love for Andrew is confirmed and deepened throughout her cancer journey. Cancer consumes her body, but it cannot claim this love or her history with Andrew. Sarah runs with her cancer, moving at a steady pace through the horrors it brings. Here is Sarah's story: the early years of her life, the diagnosis of cancer and its treatment, her beliefs about this disease, and her quest for survival.

The Early Years

Sarah was born in Manitoba. Hers was a 1950s family: mother, father, two brothers, and a sister. While life appeared "normal" to outsiders, Sarah recalls that her father was physically abusive toward her mother.

The four of us kids, we were witness to a lot of that. The four of us would be huddled in the corner just screaming and this would be going on and so it was, it was pretty traumatic and I think that affected me a lot.

Father was "master of the house." He ruled, he punished, he meted out discipline. He frightened Sarah. On one occasion Sarah and her brother came home from school to find their mother seriously injured. She had been beaten bloody by Sarah's father.

My brother and I had been out and the back door was locked. We couldn't get in. It was in the summertime and we walked into the house. He came, he heard us at the back door and unlocked it and he walked us into the house and he said, "Oh, your mother has fallen and I have to take her to the hospital." We, we went into the bedroom and there was blood everywhere — on the walls, on the bed. You know, if she fell then why is there blood on the bed and a puddle by the door and so on. So he disappeared with her to the hospital. And I was so terrified. I was very afraid of him because he was so violent.

Sarah's mother needed 65 stitches to close her head wounds. Convulsions revealed the act's savagery. Having survived the beating, Sarah's mother filed for divorce. Sarah saw her father on two later occasions and then never again. He called her when she was first diagnosed with cancer. A voice from her past. Sarah provided him with technical details, a grocery list of her tests and appointments. She was talking with a stranger.

Sarah's mother sought comfort in prescription drugs. Valium in particular provided a safe haven. Sarah's mother enjoyed the numbness

— how this medication made the sharp cuts and pain in her life dull and vague. Unused to having full responsibility for raising her children, she consulted four physicians who supplied her with the tranquilizers.

Mother was on all kinds of drugs that were counter-indicative of each other and, oh, it was just a nightmare. I remember when I was 16 phoning the doctor and, saying, "Could you please not prescribe any more drugs to my mom." I don't know where I got the nerve but I was just so terrified of what was going on. I mean I found her on the floor. We had a fire in our home because she was smoking.

A survivor, Sarah remained at home until she was 17. Her relationship with her mother became unbearable and Sarah quit school, left home, and sought a life on her own. She put herself through one year of university, but could not continue because of financial pressures. She worked for many years as an administrative assistant in a manufacturing plant, then became program manager for a sports association.

Sarah's younger brother died in a motorcycle accident when an elderly woman, drunk on sherry, made an illegal turn. Martin's body travelled a great distance through the air before it thudded down on the pavement. "He had a ruptured spleen, ruptured heart, and almost every bone in his body broken." Sarah's mother, floating along in a drug-induced haze, was unable to identify Martin's body at the hospital morgue. Sarah had to claim her brother's body. His death profoundly affected Sarah.

Sarah's first marriage was brief. Within a few months Sarah realized that she did not love her husband. Their marriage was a convenience, something expected of a woman Sarah's age. It was her ex-husband's need to control Sarah that eventually led to their divorce. "If I wanted to be controlled and manipulated and do everything I'm told then I would have stayed married to this person. I left him." Although the divorce was amicable, Sarah vowed never to marry again.

I just said, "That's it. I'm not going to meet anybody and I'm never going to get married again." I thought, "Okay, you went, entered into a relationship, you made some mistakes, you were under the misconception that everything was going to be perfect ... well it can't be and you can't be assured of that so you're never going to get married again."

And then Sarah met Andrew. "He just stumbled into my life one day." The stumble led to a falling in love. They left Canada to live in France where Andrew played soccer with the French National Team. They toured Italy and vacationed in Spain and Portugal.

Just like out of a storybook. I'd come over [to France] and take the cheapest flight and that meant to London because at the time there were no cheap flights to Paris, so I'd go to London and then I'd go to Dover and then I'd take the hovercraft or the ferry and then the train from Calais to Paris and then Andrew would meet me in Paris and we'd spend a few evenings in Paris and walk along the Champs Elysées and it was wonderful.

A fairy tale romance. Paris in the spring. They strolled down the Champs Elysées. Sarah and Andrew were in love and it was wonderful. Sarah calls Andrew "a gift." While living in Europe, she received news that her mother was deathly ill and flew back to Manitoba. Her mother's condition improved after six weeks and Sarah went back to France. Within two days of Sarah's return, her mother died. Tired of its hostage status, her mother's liver failed. Unable to fly back because of the cost, and reassured by her family that it was pointless to do so, Sarah missed the funeral and the burial. She regrets not having returned to bury her mother, to make peace with the dead. Sarah feels a lack of closure around her mother's death. It was as if her mother simply disappeared, abducted by death.

The Later Years: A Diagnosis and the Mastectomy

A runner for 15 years, Sarah notices a drop in her energy level. She cannot complete her usual distances. Persistent fatigue. This symptom, although troublesome, is sufficiently vague that it does not signify any specific health problem. At the end of October, while taking a shower, Sarah discovers a lump in her right breast. She is vigilant in protecting herself. She continually monitors her body, particularly her breasts. Her mother was diagnosed with breast cancer. Sarah knows she has to be careful.

And it was kind of shocking, because I had been aware of my family history with my mother having breast cancer, and I was being very cautious about it. Examining myself, maybe not as often as I should have, but I did go to the doctor. I had mammograms yearly and I did have the doctor examine me every six months and so when I found the lump, I was quite shocked.

How could this lump have gone undetected? Sarah's physician examined her six months ago. Two different pairs of hands palpated this breast — her physician's hands with their clinical sense, and Sarah's fingers with their intimate familiarity of her flesh. Referred to a surgeon for a biopsy, her cancer journey officially commences.

I went and saw the surgeon and he checked it over and he also looked at the mammograms and he said that 97 percent, there's a 97 percent chance that it's not cancerous, by the way the mammogram looked and by the way the mass felt to him.

The surgeon expresses optimism that the lump is not cancerous, but Sarah, uneasy about the change in her breast tissue, senses this lump may be cancerous. "I was very suspicious myself even though the doctor tried to be encouraging. Because of my family history, I've always had it in the back of my mind that it might be a problem for me one day." Sarah is prepared for cancer. She rehearses her response to a diagnosis of malignancy. She walks herself through the scenario — the doctor, the news, her tears.

Cancer. Sarah is diagnosed with breast cancer. Recognizing the tenacity of this disease and its destructive potential, she says to her surgeon, "Do what you have to do." The "doing" is a mastectomy. Sarah's choice is to remove as much breast tissue as possible. "For my own peace of mind, the more tissue they removed the safer I felt at that point."

After the mastectomy, Sarah is afraid to look at her scar line. The loss frightens her; the chest wall without her breast. "You have breasts from the time you are 13 or 14 years old, and then all of a sudden ... and it's not much different than having a hand removed." Sarah is pressured to gaze at her scar line.

I was *very* scared. I said, "Oh, I am afraid to have the dressing taken off." And the nurse said that I had to look at the scar. I had to. And that really upset me because I wanted to do this in my own time. I didn't want a deadline.

Cancer forces its way into her life and now a nurse wants Sarah to deal with it, to look at the reality present in the crimson scar. Sarah refuses to look at herself in the hospital. She waits until she is at home in the safety of her bedroom, alone. Standing at a distance from her mirror and without wearing her contact lenses, Sarah gently views her wound in the soft fuzziness of myopia.

What I found so amazing is you, like girls remember what they're like before they have breasts and you have breast tissue, like men and women have tissue, skin tissue in that area, but when they do a mastectomy, it's almost, it almost makes it concave. And that's what shocked me.

Sarah thought her chest would look like the way it had before she had breasts. When she was a girl. But the operation to remove her breast also excised muscles and other flesh, leaving her with a concave surgical site; something deep and serious. It looked much worse than she had anticipated.

Sarah hides the scar from Andrew. Seven months after her mastectomy, he catches his first glimpse of Sarah's surgical site.

I went for a physical exam and Andrew was with me. So I went and put on a gown and, this is hard for me to admit, but he's never seen me without, without anything, without any clothing on since I've had the operation. I've just been too ... I don't know ... horrified myself at the change in my body without exposing it to someone else, you know, someone you care a lot about. I didn't want to horrify him. I didn't know what kind of reaction I would get. It's pretty well called abject fear. So I changed and I said, "When the doctor comes in to examine me, are you going to look?" [chuckle] Doesn't that sound like a comment from a six year old? And he said, "Well, no. Probably you don't want me to." And I said, "Oh." And when Dr. X put me on the end of the examining table and he pulled the front of the gown down and Andrew was looking away and Dr. X addressed a remark to him and Andrew looked over and kept talking to Dr. X I knew, I knew he was looking right at me and he was examining me and I thought, "Well, I guess it's about time. It's been seven months, I mean my God, it's about time. You live with this person." I said to Andrew, I said, "You looked, didn't you?" And he said, "Yes, I did." And I said, "Well, what did you think?" And he said, "I just felt really sad. I felt very, very sad, like I wanted to make things all better for you." And he said, "I know I can't." And he was really upset by that. He wanted to come over and just make that scar go away and make me whole again.

Sarah cannot bring herself to have Andrew look at her scar. She does not want to horrify him with her disfigurement. Sarah ensures her chest is covered at all times, whether by clothing or darkness. Childlike, she asks Andrew if he will look. Sensitive to his partner's feelings he replies, "No." He looks away from Sarah. In the harsh lights of the examination room Sarah is exposed beyond nakedness, beyond the breast. With her gown pulled down she knows Andrew's eyes gaze upon her body. Andrew responds not with horror, but with great sadness. In his sadness is the recognition of what Sarah has gone through, what she has endured, what she has lost. And he would make her whole again if he could.

After her mastectomy in November, Sarah believes that her cancer is completely removed, that she is rid of it. It was contained in the amputated breast, and now it is gone. "You get this vision of, okay, there was cancer and now they've removed it."

Sarah's Beliefs about Cancer

Sarah reads extensively about cancer. She knows the latest treatment options. She learns about the medical system and alternative therapies. Influenced by her cancer heritage and what she reads, Sarah believes that genetics plays a major role in the manifestation of cancer.

Like it's genetic. You hear about these stories of people who smoked since they were 15 and they're now 85 and they're still smoking and having scotch every night and that sort of thing. And you think, they've never had cancer and yet I live a certain lifestyle [healthy] and I get it, so there's some kind of genetic weakness or failing. What makes his personal chemistry so strong that his system prevents his cells from multiplying?

She mentions poisons in the water, in the food chain, and in the air. She observes that not everyone has cancer. "That's when you get back to personal makeup." Cancer is unfair. People who smoke for years and drink heavily are often spared this disease. And yet, Sarah, who runs for her life, who watches what she eats, who is careful, develops breast cancer. She considers other factors which contribute to the development of cancer. She cites stress as an example.

Maybe it's stress, cause I've had a pretty stressful life. But then other people have had a lot more stressful lives and they don't have this cancer. So, I don't know. I think I got mine because my mother had breast cancer. That's what I think. I think it was something really genetic.

Sarah considers stress as a possible contributing factor to her own breast cancer. Upon further reflection, she reinforces her hypothesis about genetics. Her mother had breast cancer. Sarah has received the genes for cancer. It is an unwanted inheritance.

Sarah is not really certain why she developed cancer. In earnest, she searches for an explanation. "I can't die from this. I don't know what caused it. Like to hell with medical reasons, I want to know my own personal reason why I got this thing."

Taking Chemotherapy: The Quest for Survival

Even though chemotherapy frightens her, Sarah commences treatment in January 1993. She imagines chemotherapy patients as almost dead, ghostlike, and headed toward their graves.

The idea of chemotherapy was extremely scary. You envision yourself being this grey skinny ghost walking around with no hair and being really pathetic looking and feeling really bad, and perhaps just going from there to your grave.

Sarah's images are based on television shows about cancer patients and also from her own experiences with friends and family members who have undergone chemotherapy treatments. "You see all that and then it's your turn." Beyond the pallor and the weight loss, Sarah knows that chemotherapy can destroy relationships, and that some men leave their sick partners.

You don't know whether the person that you live with and cares about you is going to look at you one day and say, "You're getting skinnier and skinnier, and uglier and uglier and I'm out of here." Andrew's cousin is around the same age as I am and is a diabetic. Her husband left her just after Christmas and that's what he said to her. He said, "I'm sick of you being sick. I'm sick of you looking this way. You're getting skinnier by the day. You're getting uglier by the day and I can't take it anymore and I'm out of here."

Kept in the back of her mind, these thoughts are nonetheless troublesome. Andrew's cousin became skinny and ugly and her husband left her. She talks to Andrew about this fear. These are long, intimate, unhurried conversations of the heart. Among the inventory of fears generated by cancer is the loss of close relationships. It happens to some people. Sarah knows this.

Sarah begins to lose her shoulder-length hair in March. Initially it falls out strand by strand, then in ringworm-like clumps. The hair loss makes her look diseased. By the end of March she has little hair left. Sarah describes this period as "murky" and accompanied by many tears. "You don't realize what your hair means to you until you start having to face the fact that you're going to lose it." In retrospect, having now gone through chemotherapy, Sarah would cut her hair short and spare herself the trauma of finding ribbons of hair on her pillow in the morning. Sarah takes to wearing baseball caps to cover her bare scalp.

Getting Better: The Need to Focus on the Self

Before cancer and before chemotherapy Sarah always took care of other people's feelings. Sensitive persons often forego their own feelings in the need to care for others. Cancer changes Sarah. For the first time in her life, Sarah accords priority to herself, to her feelings, and to her own needs.

I've learned over the last six months that I've got to focus on myself. I've got to be number one. If somebody comes over and my house is a mess and that causes me stress, that's not good. If somebody comes over and this place is a mess and they care about me, then it's not an issue. I think that was one of the hardest things I found to do, was to say, "Okay, I'm number one now." I have to be number one to get through this.

Sarah directs her caring toward herself. She and Andrew develop a telephone "code." Two rings followed by a hang up and then another ring means that Andrew is calling. This ensures Sarah does not have to talk with anyone other than Andrew and that she is able to conserve her energy. "I only have enough strength to support myself right now. I can't help you. I've got to work for me and I've never been a person to do that." Sarah takes steps to reduce stress in her life.

Cancer Recurrence

Sarah's final chemotherapy treatment is scheduled for the last week of June. Her hair grows tuft-like and she no longer wears her baseball cap.

Her spirits are good. She starts to run again, something she has not done since her cancer diagnosis. She and Andrew plan a holiday together to mark the end of the treatments. Andrew and Sarah invite friends and the chemotherapy nurses to a party to celebrate the completion of her treatment, the end of cancer. On a sunny summer afternoon, Sarah rides her bike to the cancer clinic.

It was a beautiful gorgeous day. I went in and Jane [cancer nurse] said, "Well, let's give you your examination and we'll send you for chemo after." And so she examined me and she asked me to do something with my hands that I never had to do before and it was to put my hands over my head and press. And I thought, why is she asking me to do that? In all of the 14 examinations I had since January I've never had to do that. But I did it and she stood back and she was frowning. And she said, "I don't want to worry you but I need to call in Dr. X because along the scar line, I think there are two small tumours. Or they could be fibroid tissue." The doctor came in and he looked at it and he didn't say anything and then he left and he came back in about five minutes and he said, "Well, I'm not gonna pull any punches, it's cancer."

Sarah arrives at the cancer clinic anticipating liberation from her ordeal. She describes herself as being on the crest of a wave of happiness. "You're so excited about getting rid of this out of your body and walking away from all this horror scene and thinking this is the end of the siege I've been under and then you get thrown into this pit of despair." Sarah plummets from her lightness of being into a pit of darkness and despair.

The cancer nurse steps back from Sarah. She moves away — perhaps in fear or disbelief from what her fingertips have found along Sarah's scar line. While Sarah hears what the oncologist says to her, she feels as though she is far removed from the events at hand. She leaves her body. "It's almost like you're a third person at this point. You're so busy dealing with the anxiety and fear that it sounds like they're talking to you from a long ways away." The cancer nurse cries. Sarah takes this as a sign that she will die. "Why is Jane sitting there crying? I'm going to die!" Jane explains her tears: they are teardrops of anger, frustration, and the heartache of recently having a husband die of cancer. Sarah and Jane cry together, each providing comfort to the other.

Sarah cannot ride her bike back home. Upon hearing that her cancer has spread, she becomes weak and disoriented. Numbness sets in.

Her body and feelings freeze. A nurse calls a taxi for Sarah. She arrives home with the burden of telling Andrew that her cancer has spread. "Out of the whole experience, if I could have changed anything, it was having to tell Andrew." Andrew and Sarah hold each other and weep. Sorrow in the afternoon of a sunny summer day.

Sarah undergoes another biopsy. The doctor removes a piece of tissue from her scar line and places it in a specimen jar. Sarah speaks of the insult of cancer.

I think cancer's a real insult. And that was just more insulting to have to go and lay out there like a carcass and have this, this piece of you taken and sent away in a jar. I even had to carry the jar up to the lab on the fifteenth floor and look at it in the jar.

Her body, as if already dead, is stripped of flesh. Sarah carries her cancer, her burden, to the lab. While in the elevator she looks with amazement at the pink tissue as it floats innocently in the clear preservative. She is puzzled at how something this small, her rosy flesh, could cause so much pain in her life. A pathologist confirms what Sarah and her oncologist already know. The flesh in the jar and in Sarah's chest is malignant. Sarah undergoes a battery of tests: a liver scan, bone scan, chest X-ray, and blood work. Cancer has not spread beyond the scar line.

Sarah takes a new chemotherapeutic agent: adriamycin. Its potency is revealed in Sarah's nausea, vomiting, and fatigue. "I felt like I was shot in the head. I felt so terrible." Sarah spends several days in bed recuperating from the effects of the chemotherapy. Her hair falls out again. "It started right away and it's really dramatic. I'd show you but it's kind of gross." Sarah picks up the stray hairs from her clothes as if they are lint. She examines every hair in her pinched fingers. This gesture becomes a habit. She relocates the wayward hairs to the carpet. Sarah's hair drifts over her furniture, over the back of her favourite chair. It marks the territory of a person with cancer. Chemotherapy blisters her skin around the site where it enters her body. The back of Sarah's hand swells, and hard, painful lumps develop. A port, a little tube, is put in near Sarah's collarbone to save her hand veins and to ease her discomfort. Sarah receives adriamycin until the end of December.

Good news. The chemotherapy works. The tumours along Sarah's scar line shrink. They soften. Sarah's cancer may be tempered into assuming a kinder stance, a remission. Both Andrew and Sarah are encouraged by the effects of the chemotherapy.

Everything seemed really good. My blood had bounced right back up to normal — healthy levels. The doctors are only monitoring one tumour now cause the other tumour is gone, and the tumour that they first started to monitor, the large tumour had measured 1.4 centimetres and today it was between 3 and 4 millimetres in size.

Sarah's oncologist is pleased with the progress: "You're really reacting well to the chemotherapy and after such a short period of time. You're turning around really nicely. This is really positive." Sarah and Andrew are ecstatic.

Taking chemotherapy is not easy. Treating cancer comes with a cost. Sarah speaks of a decline of hope, energy, and optimism. She feels that the chemotherapy depresses her immune system and suppresses her energy.

I want to hope so much that everything's going well, I do hope that everything's going to be okay with me, but there's times when I don't feel as confident as other times and I think those times are hooked up to when I'm down from that really serious chemo treatment of the first of my cycle and I think it's all connected. It's not even like a depression. It's just like your immune system's depressed, your energy level's suppressed and so is everything else. Like your hope, your optimism, your energy .... it's all just .... like there's a huge rock on you and you have to struggle out from under that rock, push it aside and go on and rebuild again. It's like your whole soul is involved in this suppression. And that's what that chemo treatment does to me every time.

Each time Sarah begins a new cycle she experiences the side effects of chemotherapy. Her body and soul are weakened, she feels crushed by the burden. She endlessly pushes her rock only to have it roll back down upon her every few weeks. Struggling out from beneath this slab-like heaviness, Sarah rebuilds and engages in life.

But the chemotherapy ... in my heart of hearts I know why people refuse chemotherapy. This is way worse than the cancer. I mean I haven't felt a lot of the cancer. I haven't had a lot of agony and pain and that sort of thing. But the chemotherapy is unbelievable. You just feel like you don't have any desire to live, you don't have any energy, you just feel like you're dying. And that's what exactly the chemotherapy makes you feel like. It's so hard.

For Sarah, taking chemotherapy is like dying. It is worse than cancer.

Supplementing the Chemotherapy

Sarah does not rely solely on chemotherapy to treat her cancer. She uses a variety of self-treatments including visualization, herbal tea, and mega-vitamins. At night in her bed and before sleep Sarah engages in visualization to assist her body in controlling the cancer.

I think really strongly in terms of getting control. I think, okay, the thymus produces the t-cells and the bone marrow produces the b-cells and then there's the helper cells and the killer cells and what they do and which ones recognize antigens and which ones don't. And then I lay there at night and I think in those terms and I get the thymus producing the right ones for certain portions of the cancer and recognizing certain things and I get the bone marrow going. But it has to be given instructions for different parts of the body and I get those b-cells and I'm the orchestra leader. I'm the one with the brains ... they're just the stupid cells. They don't know what to do so I have to tell them what to do. Then there's little scavenger guys who go around and eat it all up. And that's what I'm working with a lot lately because I realize that as this cancer is being killed off it needs the scavengers to come and eat up that portion of the cells.

Sarah guides her cells. She orchestrates their involvement in the quest to control her cancer. T-cells, b-cells, helper and scavenger cells — Sarah has all of these cells in her mind as they float through her body. Sarah also takes a special herbal tea, slippery elm, morning and evening. During the day Sarah ingests mega-vitamins. She is careful to obtain nine hours of sleep a day and 12 hours per day on the weekends. Physicians at the cancer clinic initiate their scientifically-based medical treatment routines. Sarah follows suit and starts her own home-based remedies.

The Cancer Clinic Family

During the course of her chemotherapy Sarah befriends several fellow patients at the clinic. They receive chemotherapy treatments on the same day. Sarah speaks fondly of these people, her cancer friends. She worries when she does not see them, wonders whether they are too ill to receive chemotherapy or worse, whether they are dying.

There are three or four people I had gotten really close to. There's Richard and his wife Linda ... and I haven't seen them in two months. Margaret, another girl who was diagnosed with breast cancer and has a new baby, I hadn't seen her in about three months and I was really worried about her. And also I saw Larry who's a police officer ... well he's on disability leave right now. And then I saw Peter, a 19-year-old boy from Portage, who had a problem with his liver. I saw him today. He looks fantastic and I was just so excited to see him and we had such a good visit and all these people, like Richard, Margaret, Larry, and Peter, all these people I hadn't seen for months ... and I saw them today. It was such a wonderful day and I visited with them.

Sarah has a second family whose members bond because of a disease and its treatment. Those whose lives have become forever altered by cancer are capable of quick empathy. They are demonstrative and readily affectionate. "There's no inhibitions, you're dealing with life and death."

And then Larry dies. Sarah knew something was wrong when she saw Larry's wife without him at the cancer clinic. "I looked at her and I knew right away, I just knew." Sarah comforts Larry's wife and extends her condolences. Sarah is stunned. "I just felt like somebody had hit me in the head with a two-by-four." That same afternoon, as she completes her treatment, Sarah finds out that Margaret has also died. Grief and fear grip her.

Like to be there for your worst chemo and then to see these people die.... I came home that night and it was so, it was such a downer. I was really upset. It scared me badly too. You know how I'm so adamant about getting over this disease and handling it and coping and fighting it and everything else. This shook me to my very core and I've been, I've been unable to sleep well.

Sarah clearly sees her own mortality in the deaths of members of her cancer family. They share a collective morbidity and many are destined to a common mortality. Sarah tries to handle cancer, to fight it, but these deaths cut to the core of her being.

Viewing Life as a Person Living with Cancer

Cancer changes Sarah in many ways. Beyond her mastectomy, her exposed scalp, the nausea, vomiting, and heavy fatigue, Sarah undergoes a transformation in how she views the world. From the perspective of a person living with cancer, details of daily living become important.

Having a diagnosis with cancer is like getting a wake-up call. You really are looking at the individual snowflakes. You're looking at the rain coming down. You're smelling the air and just all the wonderful things there are and you didn't even know. You think you're enjoying life, but once you get cancer, I mean it's a whole other set of values. Everything just seems to become gilt-edged.

The world is a gilded wonder. Sarah pauses and takes in everything: snowflakes, rain, air. She captures snowflakes in her cupped hands and on her tongue. The white flakes, like winter butterflies, land on her eyelids. She views the world in amazement. She needs to take in the details before her. The ordinary becomes extraordinary. "You don't know how much time you have. Nobody does, but it's a little scarier when you've got cancer." She views the world as if through the eyes of a child. Cancer provides Sarah with a new lens. It is the wonder of the world that she sees.

Sarah also scans the obituaries to see who has died of cancer. It is a form of death voyeurism. Although embarrassed by this activity, Sarah feels she has certain rights and privileges as a person living with cancer. Monitoring the cancer death toll is one of them. "I found myself going through the obituaries looking at the bottoms to see where in lieu of flowers people were asked to donate to the Cancer Society." Sarah observes that on one Saturday, 10 of the 25 obituaries note the presence of cancer — either directly as the cause of death or indirectly as a thank-you to the staff of the cancer clinic for their care.

The Cancer Dream

Sarah has not had a nightmare since she was a child. The cancer present in her body creeps into her consciousness. Unrestricted in its associative abilities, Sarah's mind conjures up a night terror, a dream filled with horror. A cancer dream.

A really vivid dream about my cancer, but it was so bad. It was just before the finish of my last treatment on the last cycle of therapy that I was going through. I woke up at 5 in the morning and I had *the* worst nightmare. And

I'm not a nightmare person. It was so vivid I couldn't calm down for about four hours after I woke up. I was so afraid that even when I woke up, I was looking around the room, walking around, checking the doors, looking out the windows. It was a dream about a man and the man was everything that was evil. And he was coming to find me no matter where I went or what I did. And this dream went on for quite a while. This man was just slowly, methodically coming after me, looking for me, trying to find me, and finding me and discovering me, and coming towards me, and threatening me. And then I would find another avenue of escape and I would run away and get away and I would be hiding and he would find me … slowly, methodically. And he was this grey man. He was wearing a grey shirt, grey pants and grey shoes. I think he represented cancer. I have never had a dream that haunted me so badly. It was just terrifying.

Slowly and methodically an evil shadows Sarah. No matter where she tries to hide or flee, it finds her. Sarah is pursued by something displaying a cool and rational determination in its quest to locate her, to consume her. "The fear was unbelievable. I don't think I've ever been that afraid." Grey. The man in Sarah's dream is the colour of many patients taking chemotherapy. It is a colour Sarah associates with cancer.

The Body Cancer

Toward the end of September, Sarah experiences pain in her lower spine. She does not tell anyone about it. Not her oncologist, not Andrew, no one. Sarah cannot speak of what her body knows. Fear contains the message within the confines of her bones. Sarah believes the pain may be related to the new chemotherapeutic agent she has been taking. Or it may be the strain of carrying grocery bags. Her bones might be tired. She does not mention cancer, although she speaks of death.

But when I start to think about it … I was thinking about it a lot in bed the other night and I thought, "Well, I'm not afraid to die, I'm really not." I haven't been the greatest person, but I've been pretty good. The only part is, like I can't believe is, what if I have to leave? What if I have to not be here anymore? I'm just enjoying things so much. That's the thing that really bothers me. I'm not afraid of a painful death. But I don't want to leave my friends and all the fun things and stuff like that. I got really philosophical because of the aches and pains.

Cancer's destructive might is first revealed in physiology. Then it is a matter of time before it spreads beyond cells and begins to consume life. Cancer claims hopes and dreams. Most horribly, it devours the future.

It's your life flashing before your eyes. It's all the things that mean so much to you. That's the worst part because I feel I've gone through a lot of tragedies and I finally — in the last 8 to 10 years have found peace, joy, comfort, and just really enjoying life. And then this happened. I said to myself, "Well, you've had eight really nice years and that's better than none." I don't think of this often, but every once in a while when you think about your own mortality ... I thought, "Well, if something happens I guess it wouldn't be that bad now because I've had some joy out of life." And then when it [cancer] happened I thought, "Oh no. This is not enough. I want a lot more. I want a lot more years and I'm just enjoying myself too much." I'm not afraid to die, but I don't want to leave what I have.

Terrified of what the scan might show, Sarah asks Andrew to accompany her to the cancer clinic. She undergoes a bone scan in January. The results are not good. Her cancer has spread to her bones: one of her hips, the lumbar area of her spine, and a rib. The aches and pains Sarah experienced in her spine at the end of September were not related to strain, or overexertion. They were cancer taking root. The oncologist calls it "shadowing." In Sarah's cancer dream, an evil stranger shadows her: The man in grey. Sarah's nightmare comes true.

But ... the news [speaking softly and slowly]. The bone scan came back showing some spots of cancer. It has metastasized into the bones ... in three spots. So I started a brand-new chemo on Wednesday ... um ... different drugs.

Sarah is placed on vinblastine and mitomycin-C, her third treatment regimen since commencing chemotherapy in January. Such changes do not bode well for people with cancer. Chemotherapy appears incapable of stopping Sarah's cancer. Sarah, however, remains hopeful about her prognosis. "I know my chances of survival are a lot less than they were before because of this, but I know they're not zero and I can be a statistic. I can also be a statistic on the survival side of things." Sarah runs for her life.

At this point, after two chemo failures, Sarah takes control of her treatment regimen. She puts together an action plan, a cornucopia of alternative therapies. "This is the big fight!" Her plan entails consulting an herbalist and an acupuncturist, taking yoga and relaxation courses, and participating in a support group. Sarah also writes to a physician in Montreal. He treats cancer patients with nitrogen injections and he will forward these injections to a Winnipeg-based physician of Sarah's choosing. She will monitor how she progresses on the new chemotherapy for three months. If it does not appear to work, she will stop the treatments.

I'm going to take charge. I cannot wait for the medical community to do something for me. And I'm going to get the nitrogen treatments and they will help my body. I want to have them [alternative therapies] all lined up. I want to be able to reach out and call them in when I need them and when I think that I'm ready for them.

Sarah can no longer rely solely on her oncologist for help. She embarks on a new quest for a cure or at least a treatment that will keep her cancer from advancing any further. She also types up a list of anything that causes stress in her life and takes measures to eliminate as many of these stressors as possible.

Fatigue. A dense, heavy tiredness falls on Sarah. She notices a significant decrease in her energy level. "I don't know, I'm so tired all of the time. This chemo treatment really affected me." Sarah is also acutely aware that her cancer may take her life. "I do not want to die. I do not want this to threaten my life, and it is." Sarah is hospitalized for six weeks during March and early April because her cell counts drop dangerously low. Sarah nearly dies during this hospital stay. Because the chemotherapy becomes life threatening — she cannot produce enough blood cells to fight off infection — Sarah instructs the physicians to stop the treatments. She then makes exclusive use of alternative therapies.

*

Sarah died in a hospital on Saturday, June 4, 1994, with Andrew at her side.

*

I want to get married this summer and I want to get better. And, you know, I want to have a wonderful life with Andrew — I do have a wonderful life with him but I want that to continue. And I want to have my friends and family around me that I care very much about and that, that's my wish list. I don't care about anything else.

— *Sarah, November 12, 1993*

LESSONS LEARNED: SARAH'S GIFTS TO US

There are many lessons in Sarah's narrative. We learn how important it is for women to conduct breast self-exams, especially when there is a history of cancer in the family. Sarah teaches us how we must listen to our bodies and trust our own body knowledge. An intelligent person, she demonstrates how information empowers women who face breast cancer. Knowledge allows women to assume some control of their cancer care. Despite this information, Sarah also lived with fears about her cancer.

Family History of Cancer

Sarah had a family history of breast cancer. Her mother was diagnosed with breast cancer. Sarah knew she had to be vigilant and she examined her breasts for any changes or lumps. Her family history of breast cancer placed her in a high risk category.

- If you have a history of cancer in your family, discuss this with your physician. A family history of cancer generally increases your risk of cancer. Your physician may recommend specific screening techniques depending on the type of cancer in your family.

Sarah commented that perhaps she could have examined her breasts more often then she did. She was surprised when she felt a lump in her breast. The lump had grown quite large before Sarah discovered it.

- Breast self-exams (BSE) should be conducted on a regular basis. The Canadian and American Cancer Societies can direct you to where you can learn how to do BSE. A women's health clinic can also assist you.

- BSE is only effective if you actually *perform* it.

- Some women who are at high risk of developing breast cancer may also undergo yearly mammograms.

Learning how to perform a breast self-exam and then conducting it on a regular basis may save the lives of many women or contribute to more years of survival after a diagnosis of cancer. Women who regularly perform breast self-exams can detect even minor changes in their breasts. Mammography — a low dose X-ray of the breast — works best with less dense breast tissue, typically women over the age of 50. High risk women aged 40 to 49 or younger should consult their health care provider about having mammography screening.

Listening to Your Intuition

When Sarah discovered this lump in her breast, she sensed that it was cancer. The surgeon she consulted encouraged her not to worry. He suggested the lump was likely not cancerous. Sarah eventually received confirmation of her suspicions. The biopsy revealed that the breast lump was cancerous.

- Every breast lump must be viewed with suspicion and caution until a definitive diagnosis is made by a physician.

You may find that sometimes physicians and other health care providers, in their efforts not to alarm women, suggest that a lump is "probably nothing." The more sensitive and less damaging observation would be, "There is a lump in your breast. A biopsy will reveal whether the lump is cancerous or not." Because Sarah knew intuitively that this lump was cancer, she was not surprised when the biopsy proved the surgeon wrong. Women are often told, "Don't worry. The lump is most likely benign!" and then they are notified that the lump is cancerous after all. Trust, an essential element in the relationship between patient and physician, is breached when such bold, hopeful statements are not substantiated. Although these statements provide temporary relief, they can be harmful in the long term. Erosion of trust and a loss of confidence in one's physician should not characterize the beginning of the cancer journey. Of course, every woman hopes that the lump in her breast is not cancer. However, assuming cautious optimism is prudent.

Journey at Your own Pace

Sarah journeyed at her own pace. She looked at her mastectomy scar only when she was ready. A nurse pressured her to "deal with it." Sarah was expected to look at her scar line and face the reality that her breast was gone.

- As a person with cancer, do not let other people — whether family, friends, or health care providers — push you into doing something you do not wish to do. Resisting others sometimes requires courage and fortitude. And you may need others to back you up as you seek to journey at your own pace.

- Viewing your mastectomy scar for the first time may be frightening. Some women take "small steps" toward looking at their surgical sites. Over a period of several days they gradually progress from looking down at their chest wall when the dressing is changed, to looking at themselves in the bathroom mirror. Let the nursing staff know what your wishes are in terms of seeing your mastectomy site. It is your choice as to how and when you will finally examine your scar.

- You can obtain pictures of what a mastectomy site looks like — before your surgery. This can help prepare you for the shock of seeing your chest wall without the presence of your breast.

- Some women request reconstructive surgery at the time of their mastectomies. Talk to your physician about what process is right for you.

Although pressured by a nurse, Sarah refused to examine her scar line until she was ready. She waited until she was in the safety and comfort of her home before she looked at her operative site. Sarah took out her contact lenses and then stood at a distance from the mirror. She walked slowly toward her image, blurred in the fuzziness of short sightedness, and finally saw her chest wall without her breast. Viewing the mastectomy scar is a painful moment; Sarah ensured that viewing her scar was done on her terms, at her own pace.

Learning about Breast Cancer

Because Sarah read extensively about breast cancer, she was able to make informed decisions about her treatment. Sarah could never get enough information about breast cancer. She empowered herself through knowledge.

- If you want to participate in decisions about your breast cancer, then you need to be informed. Become your own advocate — find out as much as you can about breast cancer.

- Information about the treatment of breast cancer is available from a variety of sources. You can contact the Canadian or American Cancer Societies about existing resources. The Internet is a particularly helpful resource. Located on the Internet are women's own accounts of their breast cancer experiences including pictures of their operative sites. You can search for "cancer" in general, or narrow your search by a particular cancer type — breast cancer, prostate cancer, lung cancer, etc.

- On the Internet, The National Cancer Institute (NCI) offers "PDQ Information Packages" for breast cancer patients and physicians. You may wish to read both of these packages in terms of learning about the treatment of breast cancer.

- Some excellent web sites on the Internet include:

  National Cancer Institute: CancerNet Cancer Information
  http://cancernet.nci.nih.gov/icichome.htm

  WWW Cancer
  http://www.arc.com/cancernet/cancernet.html

  American Cancer Society
  http://www.cancer.org

  Canadian Cancer Society
  http://www.cancer.ca

Sarah decided not to opt for a lumpectomy. Rather, she requested a mastectomy. Given her mother's diagnosis with breast cancer, she wanted her entire breast removed. Sarah felt more secure undergoing this extensive surgical procedure.

Fears Associated with Breast Cancer

Sarah experienced fear as a woman living with cancer. Sarah was frightened that with her body disfigured by cancer, her partner would leave her. This had happened to other women she knew. Sarah spoke with Andrew about this particular fear. She needed to know how he felt about the changes to her body — the losses of her breast, her hair, and her weight.

- Given the impact that cancer has on our bodies and our lives, people living with cancer usually experience fear.

- Your fears need to be addressed. Talking about them sometimes helps. Getting information can also be of value. Our fears can be eased when we understand why we have them.

- Trying to protect family members from the realities of the cancer experience (i.e., hiding your mastectomy scar), may prove effective in the short term, but can be destructive in the long term. It also takes more energy to sustain this protection and, as a person living with cancer, you need this energy for other things.

- With the loss of a breast, women can have fears of rejection and the disintegration of intimate relationships. Sometimes these fears are well founded and counselling may be needed to ensure the survival of relationships. Despite these efforts, some relationships will fail. It is important to discuss your fears with those who love and care for you. Ignoring your fears or hoping they will go away will not lead to their resolution.

- Support groups for spouses may help husbands or partners come to terms with their own fears concerning breast cancer. Some men may be more comfortable taking part in Internet-based support groups.

♦ Keep the lines of communication open with those whose lives intimately intersect with your life.

Sarah was able to talk to Andrew about her fears. She set aside specific time to speak with him about her concerns. They spoke during the quiet of the evening, taking the phone off the hook so as to not be disturbed. Some women who fear their partners may leave them are unable to talk about this. Rather than ignore the possibility that Andrew might leave her, Sarah chose to directly deal with this fear.

Sarah could not talk about all of her fears. She would not tell anyone about the pain in her spine. She bore this pain in silence, alone and too frightened to consider what the pain meant. It was four months before her bone scan picked up metastases to her spine and ribs.

♦ Fear that your cancer has spread can immobilize you. Pain is an indicator that something is wrong. Although we may fear the worst, reporting the presence of pain or other symptoms is important. Your physician needs to know this information to take appropriate action and provide you with the best care possible.

♦ Fear can make you suffer in silence and turn your cancer journey into a profoundly lonely experience.

♦ Keeping "secrets" from your physician undermines your relationship and erodes trust, especially when this information can have an impact on your survival.

Talking with someone might have eased some of Sarah's burden associated with this fear. Had Sarah shared the information about her pain, her physician could have taken steps to alleviate it. Silenced by fear, Sarah suffered with this secret for four months.

Be Kind to Yourself: Letting Go of Things

Always giving, Sarah began to focus on herself for the first time in her life. Living with cancer demanded she take care of herself. For her, this meant letting go of certain things in her life. She learned not to worry about whether her home was spotless. Giving up the need to keep her home immaculate freed up energy for Sarah. She then directed this energy to living with cancer.

- Many people start to take care of themselves for the first time in their lives once they are diagnosed with cancer. Cancer demands attention to the self and spending time on yourself is part of the cancer journey.

- Reassess your priorities around the home. Trying to maintain a certain standard of cleanliness without your usual energy levels can be frustrating at best and cause you to be extremely fatigued at worst. This is counter-productive to supporting the internal body resources you need to devote to your healing and health.

- Encourage family members to help with household chores. Changing roles within the family can be difficult, but with encouragement and guidance family members can adapt.

- Some women organize "cleaning bees" or "cooking bees" and have friends come in and help out for an afternoon. The company and the work accomplished can do wonders to lift the spirit. Moreover, work around the house gets done.

- If you can afford it, have a cleaning person come in once a month or every couple of weeks. If you cannot stand having a less than perfect home environment, this may be well worth the investment.

Sarah took great delight in pointing out what she had not accomplished in her home. The dishes were not done, the kitchen floor was not swept, and the laundry pile was higher than ever before. She directed her time and energy to other things like her relationship with her partner. Sarah also encouraged Andrew to complete household tasks.

Protecting Yourself from Intrusions

Sarah and Andrew developed a secret telephone code. This limited intrusions into their lives. Sarah would not answer the phone during the afternoon unless she knew it was Andrew. The answering machine recorded all other phone calls. Sarah did not want to be disturbed by anyone during the day — except Andrew. She did not want to be interrupted while she meditated, slept, soaked in the tub, or read.

- Setting aside rest time and quiet time for yourself, especially during chemotherapy and radiation treatments, is necessary. Sometimes friends and family members call in large numbers, creating stress and taxing your energy. Take action to protect your rest periods.

- Don't be afraid to let people know that you have to limit your phone conversations to a specific length of time. You may decide you only wish to talk with people about 5 or 10 minutes. Have a clock by the telephone and let people know when you have reached your limit.

- Ask friends to call in advance of visiting to ensure that the time is convenient for you. Again, limit visits to a reasonable amount of time. You may find that on some days you have more energy and desire a longer visit. Alternately, don't be concerned that you may only feel like visiting for a few minutes on other days. There may be days that you may not want *any* visitors.

- Fatigue, as a consequence of chemotherapy or radiation therapy, requires that you consider the following: resting frequently, prioritizing activities (what you must do versus what would be nice to do), and working smart by reducing the energy required to complete tasks.

Sarah made a list of all the stressful things in her life, including people. She then set about eliminating as many of these as possible. This was another energy conserving tactic that proved successful for Sarah.

The Uncertainty Associated with Cancer

Cancer is characterized by uncertainty and an emotional rollercoaster ride. Unfortunately, Sarah believed that her last chemotherapy session heralded the end of her cancer. In reality, it was during this appointment that she found out her cancer had spread along her scar line. Cautious optimism may be the best policy regarding the treatment of cancer.

- Never make assumptions about your cancer treatment. Ask questions concerning the effectiveness of treatments given the stage of your cancer at the time of diagnosis. Ask your physician about the chances of a recurrence or the effectiveness of this particular treatment approach. Having some idea of treatment success rates can prepare you for possible outcomes during your own treatment experience.

♦ Having an understanding of your treatment approach may help you be hopeful but also realistic.

♦ Cautious optimism and hope, and not the certainty of success, may help to protect you from potential anguish generated by any treatment protocols that are not successful.

♦ Ask your physician what will happen should your prescribed treatment "fail" or is found to be ineffective. Find out what "Plan B" your physician might initiate or what options are then available to you.

Sarah assumed that her mastectomy and chemotherapy treatments would cure her. Her certainty caused her anguish when reality clashed with her beliefs. She had planned a party and invited her friends and the chemotherapy nurses to celebrate the end of her cancer. The ecstasy and excitement of being cured of cancer were dashed in the time it took for the nurse to run her fingers along Sarah's scar line. With a more cautious approach to cancer, Sarah might have spared herself some of this suffering. She also attended the cancer clinic alone that day.

♦ It is probably wise to have someone accompany you to the cancer clinic. Although some people might prefer to go alone, having someone who cares for you there at the clinic can make the journey easier — especially if the news is not good.

It was traumatic for Sarah to receive the news of her recurrence while alone at the clinic. In retrospect, having Andrew with her would have provided Sarah with much-needed support. Sarah was so distressed upon learning of her recurrence that she was unable to ride her bike and had to take a taxi home.

The Use of Alternative Therapies

Alternative treatment therapies or complementary therapies appealed to Sarah. She eventually became disillusioned with medicine; the treatment failures and the side effects of her chemotherapy left her seeking other ways of healing. Sarah mobilized a host of nontraditional treatments. Although these did not cure her cancer, they permitted Sarah to exercise some control over her situation. Alternative therapies enabled her to actively participate in her cancer care. Things were no longer just done to Sarah. She was actively involved in healing her body.

♦ The potential value of alternative treatment modalities has recently been recognized with the commitment of national research dollars both in Canada and the United States.

♦ Some physicians, families, and friends remain sceptical about alternative treatments, but approve of the use of these therapies in conjunction with biomedical treatments. What you *want* or *believe* is more important than what others think.

♦ Let your physician know what alternative treatments you are using — and the effect you feel they are having.

♦ Talk to people who have used alternative therapies to find out about their experiences.

Rebirth in the Cancer Experience

As a woman living with breast cancer, Sarah began to appreciate the wonder of life. Most of us take our lives and our worlds for granted. Cancer often changes our perception of the world and our stance in it. Sarah saw things as if for the first time. Each season brought marvellous things to her eyes: snowflakes, the winter sky, spring rain, the majestic elm trees.

♦ Cancer is a difficult disease to live with. It is fraught with suffering. However, living with cancer can afford us profound insight about life, love, and ourselves. Cancer can alter our consciousness and our being in the world.

- Because cancer can threaten our existence, reflecting upon this situation can change what we see in the world and the way we see these things.

- For some people, cancer is a wake-up call for life and living. They are reborn in the sense that life becomes more sharply focused. Life becomes more precious. Taking stock and setting priorities are common among cancer patients. This includes "cutting to the chase" and figuring out what is important in one's life.

Sarah experienced life differently while living with cancer. She understood the importance of love in her life. She realized that her partner loved her deeply and without reservation. Sarah took stock of the love in her life. Seeing the world in its amazing detail, its wonderment, and truly knowing love were nurturing to Sarah.

Sarah loved laughter. Her humour shone through the cancer atrocities. Because of the gravity of so many things surrounding cancer, Sarah saw the need to use laughter and humour to survive this disease. Sarah filled rooms with laughter. She lifted her own spirits and the morale of others through her sincere use of humour.

Sarah offered us many lessons as we journeyed with her. She reinforced the need to pay attention to family history in relation to breast cancer, and the need to regularly perform breast self-exams. She also helped us understand that everyone journeys with cancer at their own pace. As a woman who wanted to be involved in decisions about her treatment, Sarah read extensively about cancer. Gaining knowledge about cancer empowered Sarah. She was able to have a say in her cancer experience. Despite her knowledge, Sarah had many fears about her breast cancer. We learned from Sarah that talking about these fears can help tame them. One source of fear was the uncertainty associated with cancer. Sarah showed us that cautious optimism and hope help us live with the uncertainty of cancer. One way in which Sarah dealt with her uncertainty was to make use of alternative therapies. These therapies permitted Sarah to impose some order and control on the chaos generated by her cancer.

Sarah taught us about the possibility of rebirth in the cancer experience. Cancer afforded Sarah profound insight about her life and the love present in her life. Cancer served as a wake-up call for her. Stricken with a life-threatening disease, Sarah became more fully alive.

She had the opportunity to determine the priorities in her life and devote time and energy to them. Sarah also discovered that Andrew loved her unconditionally. Theirs was a deep and abiding love, beyond the torments of cancer. Sarah lived each day as a gift. She observed radiance in the ordinary and recognized that she was surrounded by something greater than herself.

6

MADELINE

LIVING ON TRUST: BREAST CANCER

MADELINE'S BLACK HAIR is cropped short to her scalp. Her lips are bloodless, her face white. Cancer and chemotherapy treatments have faded her features. Set in this pale background are Madeline's large, kind, expressive, brown eyes. Beneath them are deep black rings. These contrasts expose the seriousness of her situation.

Madeline is soft spoken and petite. She grimaces as she walks. Breast cancer has metastasized to her hip joints. She favours her left hip and left leg as she leans on a black metal cane. Diagnosed with breast cancer almost nine years ago at the age of 33, Madeline has outlived her physician's prediction of death-by-cancer by five years. She attributes her survival to the Lord. Madeline is a woman of faith. She places her life in God's hands. Faith, trust, and love of God provide her with strength, courage, and hope on her cancer journey.

Madeline, her husband Klaus, and their three teenage sons live in a middle class neighbourhood. Their split-level home and yard are neat and tidy. Klaus's gardening has produced a mass of flowers surrounding their home. When Madeline was able to work, she was a cashier in a large grocery store chain.

Madeline's story is about enduring metastatic breast cancer. She is besieged by a disease that will not stop in its pursuit of her body, her life. Consumed by cancer, Madeline's faith in God grows proportionately and in tandem with the advance of her cancer.

The Early Years

Madeline was born in a small town in rural Manitoba, the third of five daughters. Twenty-one years separates the oldest and youngest sisters. Madeline's father was a farmer and she recalls walking through wheat fields, her hands dipping into a sea of grain. She speaks of an unrestricted childhood on the plains, of moving freely under a blue prairie sky.

We were free to come and go. We were out in the fields. We were out in the dugouts, like all over the place. But you never thought of harm coming to you. We used to go on 20-mile bike rides over the fields and dirt roads and stuff. It was a great way to grow up.

Madeline met her future husband in grade four. They attended the same one-room school house. "I remember when I saw him and I thought, 'Oh I like him.'" She and Klaus began dating when they were 17. This year marks their twenty-second wedding anniversary. They have three sons: Jason, 19; John, 17; and, Jeremy, 16. Madeline describes them as "good boys."

The Mastectomy and Chemotherapy

Madeline sensed that she was destined for cancer, that one day she would be diagnosed with breast cancer. This feeling was not based on family history, rather it was Madeline's fear of cancer which tempted its occurrence in her body. Sometimes things dreaded do come true.

It was the beginning of February and there had been a program on TV about breast cancer and I said to my husband, "You know, I bet you some day I'm going to get that." Because it scared me. And he said, "Don't be so silly. Don't say something like that." Well, a couple of months later I found a lump.

Madeline had experienced pain in her right breast for many years. Concerned about this pain and its possible meaning, her physician said that it was nothing. "I had pain in that breast and he said, 'Well, there's nothing there. There's nothing there. There's nothing there.'" Madeline repeats the physician's denial of her concern three times, with a tone of disbelief and an edge of anger. Madeline knew something was terribly wrong with her breast, but she could not convince her physician. Breast pain not verifiable by science does not, it seems, exist. She discovers a granite lump in her breast at the end of February 1985. It has form and substance. Something is there.

I found a lump and I mean it was the size of a plum. It wasn't like a little tiny one. And I checked often. I checked more than once a month and the lump scared me because I thought, "Whoa, this wasn't here like a little while ago." It was the weekend and on Monday I phoned right away.

Stone fruit. A plum-sized mass had grown deep in Madeline's breast. How could this be? Madeline examined herself frequently, and her physician had just conducted a breast exam four months previously. Madeline was shocked at how quickly the lump had grown.

Madeline is advised to monitor this lump. Her family physician attempts to calm her fears. He states that at 33 she is too young to have cancer, and alternative hypotheses are formulated. The lump might have its origins in her menstrual cycle. "Come back after your period, sometimes these things disappear." Madeline completes her menstrual cycle, but this "thing" in her breast does not disappear. Her family physician then goes on holidays for two weeks, further delaying her diagnosis. Upon his return, Madeline learns that her mammogram indicates the presence of a growth. Madeline is certain the cancer had spread beyond her breast.

I could feel how it was spreading and it was in my armpit. I didn't know that at the time but when they did the operation they took lymph nodes from the armpit and they said 9 out of 10 had cancer in them so obviously I'm going to have to go for chemo.

Madeline undergoes a mastectomy of her right breast. The surgery proceeds smoothly and she does not experience any complications. Chemotherapy, however, is quite a different matter.

Madeline describes her ordeal with chemotherapy as "wicked." She has no idea what to expect, but quickly learns about the side effects and full fury of antineoplastic drugs. Unrelenting nausea and vomiting strike Madeline. Wave after sickly wave empties her stomach. She retches uncontrollably.

I was so sick it was unreal. I mean I had no idea what to expect. I went for chemo and I was fine. I came home and a couple of hours passed. No big deal and boy I guess this isn't going to bother me ... and all of a sudden I just started throwing up and that was it! I threw up for hours and then there was nothing there. You're just heaving and heaving and heaving.

She loses several kilograms in five days. When the chemotherapy nurse calls to assess how she is managing, Madeline states she is fine.

"I didn't know that this wasn't normal." When she returns to the cancer clinic, the staff become aware of her severe response to the drugs. The oncologist reduces the strength of her medication. Despite this decrease, Madeline is bedridden for two weeks after each chemotherapy treatment. "I would just be starting to feel better and then it was time for another round." These chemo cycles continue for 12 months. Madeline returns to her work as a cashier in a grocery store. She is determined not to permit cancer to destroy her life. She wants to live as normally as possible.

I went back to work. My arm really hurt, it hurt. And I thought, "I am getting that arm to work here. There is no way that I'm not working that arm."
I got full movement back and I did everything I had done before. I'm
basically a go-getter. Like I fight. I'm not ready to sit back and say, "Okay,
I can't do this anymore." You try and keep things as normal as you can.

Madeline describes herself as a fighter. She is tenacious in her will to survive the cancer. When she received her diagnosis, Madeline sobbed uncontrollably as she walked home from the physician's office. "That was about the last time I cried." No more tears are permitted during the course of her cancer journey. Madeline carries on with life, with living. Supporting Madeline in her fight against cancer is her Lord and Saviour. Madeline is a woman of great faith.

We're going to pick ourselves up and we're going to carry on with life and
we're going to make the best of this and that's basically what we did. I
should say that I have a very strong faith in the Lord. He has seen me
through this whole thing. And it's been 8 years and I know that without
Him there is no way that I would still be here.

Nine years after the initial diagnosis she continues to fight cancer. Her faith becomes stronger, her convictions growing more deeply than the cancer. It is the Lord's work.

Madeline's Beliefs about Causation

When first diagnosed with cancer, Madeline's physicians asked her a number of questions. She recalls questions about the age at which she commenced menstruation and the age at which she gave birth to her first child. Madeline reflects on the possible "causes" of breast cancer.

"I'm thinking, Okay, this is what they're saying — this and this and this, but I didn't have that." The risk factors the physicians present do not apply to Madeline.

Where does it [cancer] come from? I don't know. It's hard to say. Sometimes, I wonder, I didn't breastfeed my kids. Like to me that didn't appeal to me whatsoever. And um, of course at that time they would give you shots to dry up the milk and sometimes I think, well maybe that wasn't such a good idea. But who knows.

Madeline suggests that her cancer may have its roots in her decision not to breastfeed her infants. Although uncertain, she also attributes an injection to "dry up the milk" as a possible cause. Upon further reflection, Madeline identifies that her cancer is a part of God's plan. God has His reasons for Madeline's cancer, but she does not know what these reasons might be.

The Later Years: Breast Reconstruction and the Advance of Cancer

In keeping with her attempts to normalize her life, Madeline requests plastic surgery. Two years after her mastectomy, Madeline has reconstructive surgery. It takes five surgical procedures to restore her operative site. A skin-flap grafted from her abdomen is reshaped into a new breast. There are complications. Several months after her surgery and to her horror, Madeline discovers a lump in the reconstructed breast. Painful, the lump frightens her. A biopsy reveals a benign cyst. After a seven-month wait Madeline's breast reconstruction is finally completed. The reconstructed breast is smaller, so Madeline has a reduction of her left breast. She wants her breasts to be the same size. Madeline's breasts are still not symmetrical after the reduction — the left breast remains much larger than the right.

It was still too big and I said, "Is it going to stay this big? Is it swollen?" And he [the plastic surgeon] said, "Why? Do you want it smaller than that?" I said, "Well, yeah. I thought this was the whole idea of this. I'm going through all this agony and what for?" He says, "Well women are never the same size on both sides." It didn't work out the way I thought it would. It still aggravates me. I mean there are still days that I look at myself and I think, that is so stupid, that makes me so angry. Like I want this redone. But with everything else I'm going through, it's a minor thing right now. I can't consider it right now. Like why don't they listen to what you're saying?

Madeline is angry and upset about the plastic surgery. It did not work out the way she thought it would. She wants to look "normal" after her mastectomy, but after five operations she views herself as maimed. Moreover, for the second time in her cancer experience, a physician did not listen to what Madeline was saying.

Madeline is cancer free for the five years between 1985 and 1989. "I was feeling great, I was doing good." In December 1989, Madeline experiences a problem with her right eye. She is diagnosed with diplopia, double vision. She loses her depth perception and begins to stumble while walking. In January 1990, Madeline consults her oncologist who then refers her to an ophthalmologist. Over a period of seven months she is examined by eight different specialists. "Nobody was willing to say what it was." It is cancer. Madeline is then placed on tamoxifen, a cancer drug, in September 1990.

And then when they put me on the tamoxifen, it started taking care of the pain … gradually, like it didn't come overnight or anything. After a month I went back to work. The tamoxifen was working and my eye … all of a sudden I could read. Hey, I can see with this eye.

With her vision still somewhat blurred, Madeline trips on the front porch and breaks her ankle in July 1991. She requires surgery. Pins and screws are inserted to hold the fractured bones together. Just when Madeline begins to bear weight, she feel pains in her back. "I went to the doctor and had a bone scan and of course it was worse. The cancer was in my bones, in my spine." In December 1991, Madeline commences chemotherapy. During this time, she receives chemotherapy over a period of two weeks which is then followed by a two-week reprieve. This cycle repeats itself over eight months. Because she is unable to work, Madeline and her family experience financial difficulties.

So that's a long haul, that's a long haul. And the medication wasn't cheap, but mind you, you can get that back after a while, but in the meantime you're not working. You've only got one pay cheque coming in. That was the other thing — the hassle I had with the insurance company was just unreal. You've got to send a form in every month saying, "No, you can't work yet. No you can't work yet. No you can't work yet." Then that ran out. Then I had to go on unemployment benefits. Sick pay. That's even worse. They just do not believe that you're sick. Of course, every form you fill out you get charged. And they don't stop sending forms. So finally the unemployment ran out. Then I had to apply for Canada Pension disability. Well that took seven months before I got anything from there and in the meantime, you're living on Visa. You're paying for groceries on your Visa. It was hard emotionally. Like just mentally, how are we going to pay for this? And that's hard too, on top of everything else. That's really tough.

The Progression of Cancer: Erosion of the Body

It is June 1993, and Madeline does not feel well. She claims it is the "cancer acting up again." Malevolent behaviour. Cancer spreads to her hips and eats at the joints. Madeline undergoes five radiation treatments and commences another round of chemotherapy, which induces nausea and vomiting. She is dreadfully sick for two months. "I began throwing up June the first and didn't stop throwing up until the end of July." Walking becomes increasingly painful. The pain and nausea are unbearable, and Madeline seeks medical attention at the emergency department of a large hospital on a Saturday evening.

We went to the emergency department and of course Dr. X [the oncologist] wasn't there, so you try to give them a nine-year history in five minutes and they gave me Tylenol 3 which does not agree with me. That did absolutely nothing, nothing for the pain. When they say "writhing in agony" I know what that's exactly like. So finally they gave me a shot of Demerol. And that was wonderful because it took care of the pain, [but] by the time I got home the medication had stopped working.

Madeline cannot bring herself to go back to the hospital. Her experience in the emergency department left her traumatized and without long-term relief from her bone pain. On Sunday morning she calls the emergency department — her nausea and pain are insufferable. She is advised to try another medication which she just happens to have in her bathroom medicine cabinet. "It didn't work either." Madeline waits out the weekend and consults her oncologist on Monday morning.

He put me on morphine and they found out that didn't agree with me — that worked against me too. We later found out that all the pain killers were causing my nausea. They're giving me pain killers. They're giving me stuff for the nausea and nothing is working. It's just making me feel more nauseated. I lost 20 pounds in a couple of weeks because I just couldn't eat. I couldn't keep anything down. But I just felt, just let me die. Like I don't care anymore. Just let me die. This is enough already. I had no energy. I had nothing. I was just, just deathly ill. I just looked horrible. I was just white. It is horrible when you have 24-hour nausea. You cannot get rid of it. You try to think about something else and it's just there. It's just there, it's just there. It doesn't go away.

Madeline's nausea and pain spiral out of control. It is a physiological gridlock. She cannot eat and the medication she takes to ease her pain feeds her nausea. Her situation is torturous and she becomes despondent. She laments for an end to her ordeal: "Just let me die." Deathly ill, she is reduced to a state of nothingness — a body in the throes of relinquishing the self. "I had no energy. I had nothing." Desperate for relief from her nausea, Madeline stops taking her pain medication. "I didn't care. I'll live with the pain and it can't be any worse than this." Pain over nausea. It is a forced choice. The nausea slowly eases, but it is not until the end of July 1993 that Madeline is able to keep food in her stomach.

Madeline begins to lose her strength, her stamina. Like the colour draining from her face, she becomes a lighter shade of herself. Less substantial. Her vigour is slowly consumed by the cancer.

I think what bothers me most is like I've always, like physically I've always been a strong person. I arm wrestled my boys and they couldn't beat me. It was usually a draw but I've always been physically strong. When I want to do something I do it. I can't do that anymore and I think that's one of the things I find the hardest. I have to be dependent on someone else to do things for me. I've gotten to a point, well I cannot do it today. I will do this tomorrow, but tomorrow I may wake up and feel really rotten and I won't do anything. I can't plan ahead anymore. It's a day-by-day thing.

Forced dependency. Madeline must now rely on others. They must do things for her and to her. She cannot plan ahead. The morning may not bring a reprieve from her weakness, but a worsened physical state. The promises of a new day can be broken for people living with cancer.

Cancer and God

Madeline states that she will not completely understand why she developed cancer until she is in heaven. Things that happen on earth cannot be fully comprehended and Madeline's cancer is one of these things. Heaven holds the promise of absolute truth.

God doesn't make mistakes. So obviously there is a reason for this [cancer]. I don't know what it is. I've heard a lot of people say, "I don't know how you can handle this." And yet they see that somebody else's faith will be strengthened by seeing how mine is strengthened and how I can deal with it. It has strengthened my own faith because I see over and over and over how He helps me and where He helps me and how I can get through things. If I didn't know there was somebody else with the power looking after me, then there would be no hope. When all medical things are done that can be done and there is nothing else left ... you know there is still somebody that has control. And I totally believe that 100 percent. I'm in His hands.

God does not make mistakes. Cancer is not a biological error, a quirk of physiology. That Madeline has cancer is part of something divine, part of God's larger plan. "The Lord doesn't give you things bigger to deal with than what you can handle." Madeline is not frightened of cancer or its destructive power, its will to hurt. She is cradled in God's loving hands, protected and cared for. Whether she lives or dies is up to God. Madeline's cancer strengthens her faith and she submits to God's will.

The stronger your faith is the more willing you are to leave it with God and He will look after it. I can't do this, God. You said you would look after me. I'm leaving this with you. I'm trusting you with this and I'm not going to worry about it anymore.

She trusts God completely. Madeline is calm. She does not overtly exhibit fear of any kind. There is an aura of serenity about her. Death does not frighten Madeline. She knows that heaven awaits her. Yet, the thought of leaving her husband and her boys "behind" causes her concern.
I love my husband. I love my family. I love my cats. I just, I just love being here. I don't want to leave my kids behind. I want to be there for them. It just bothers me that I may not see my children grow up. What's going to happen to them? Death doesn't bother me. Life after death is gonna be,

I mean it's a 100 percent improvement over what we've got here. There's no doubt about that. I'm not scared to die, I don't want to die just yet. Everybody has to die and I have no trouble dealing with that, but maybe not just yet.

Faith and an intimate trust in God permit Madeline to transcend cancer. She knows what awaits her upon her death — the Elysium Fields, the Promised Land, Heaven. But Madeline is not beyond the sting of death, the love for her husband and children makes the thought of death difficult for her.

Madeline brings her cancer struggles to God with faith and love. He will take care of her and things will unfold as they should. "I don't have to try and figure it out. I don't have to try and find the solution."

The relationship just gets better because you just, you see what He's done for you and what He can do.... Your faith just gets deeper and "Well God, I can't handle this. This is in your lap and I'm going to forget about it." That's what He says to do. You're supposed to bring your problems to Him and He will take care of it.

Madeline offers her cancer burdens to God.

Surviving Cancer: A Miracle

Madeline views her survival as a miracle and a testimony of God's love for her. In 1989, she asked her oncologist how long she had to live. He stated, "three years." Five years beyond the three, Madeline has not succumbed to cancer.

You know miracles are still possible. And that's why I feel ... well, it's been eight and a half years and I'm still here. I keep on plugging away. I was so sick these two months this summer. Man, why is this taking so long? There's time when you feel like "I'm never going to get better. This is just worse and worse and worse." And I was at a point where I don't really care if I died. But that's the easy way out. You've just got to hang in there.

God has permitted her to live, but Madeline reveals that surviving cancer is not easy. God does not spare Madeline from cancer hardships. Even believers are ravaged by this disease. Madeline chooses to "hang in there" and accept what God brings her. It is an arduous journey. She is careful to explain, however, that she is not passive about her cancer. "That doesn't mean that I can't do what's in my power to do. It's not like I'm going to say, 'No I'm not going to have chemo because God's looking after me.'" Madeline makes use of everything that the cancer clinic has to offer to treat her cancer. She trusts her life to the Lord, but "He has no problem with us using what's available for us, but still putting our trust in Him for the rest." Madeline fights her cancer with conviction.

Members of her congregation, her church family, pray for Madeline. She attests to the power of collective prayer. God has heard the prayers of these supplicants and Madeline's cancer is now quiet in her body. She takes comfort in knowing that others are praying for her.

Just knowing that people are praying for you, it's just like knowing there are loving arms around you. Even when they're not here, you know people care.

Embraced by the loving arms of prayer, Madeline is consoled and cared for by her church family. Another source of strength. Madeline's name and her sickness are entered into a book of prayer petitions. The petitions are written in a manner that affords documentation of the intercessions; the power of prayer, the work of the Lord.

And the thing is, the way we write them [the prayers] down … has to be in a way that you can see whether they are or whether they are not answered. Not just something general so that you'll never know well maybe it is or maybe it isn't.

Prayers that are answered are highlighted in pink. Some prayers take time to be answered. Madeline's petition is there, the cobalt-blue ink bleeding into a flourescent pink background. God hears. He answers her prayers.

The Advance of Cancer

Weariness descends upon Madeline in September 1993. She feels tired and without energy. Walking up a flight of stairs makes her short of breath. "I'm huffin' and puffin' and it's like I'm gonna die and this is not normal." Sleep does not relieve this state of extreme fatigue. Madeline wakes up tired.

When I got up this morning I was so pooped. I didn't get dressed until almost noon. I just sat there and sat there and thought, "Oh I've got to get up, I've got to get up." I had absolutely zero energy and I still can't get that.

It takes her three hours to clean a shower stall. This is the only physical activity she can manage during the day. She cannot complete a task without taking frequent breaks, she must lie down.

At the end of September the chemotherapy treatments are stopped. Madeline's blood counts fall dangerously low. She receives two units of blood at the cancer clinic. A severe pain develops in Madeline's right arm. It consumes her.

This arm. Ahhh, this arm. I don't think I've ever had such bad pain. Sunday afternoon the pain started in my arm and it just didn't go away. Sometimes it was like lightning bolts. All I could think of was pain, pain, pain. You couldn't focus your mind on anything else. I didn't sleep at night. Are the rest of my days going to be like this? It's only pain, pain, pain. I've had enough. I don't want anymore. The cancer nurse said, "No. We have to get rid of the pain and get you back on your feet."

Pain, pain, pain. Words cannot convey what she experiences and Madeline can only repeat the word "pain" to describe her plight. In addition to her pain, Madeline loses strength in her arm and hand and must use her left hand. Another loss, another change. Her oncologist orders tests to determine the source of the pain. Scans of Madeline's brain, her axillary region, and abdomen are taken. A consult with a neurologist is arranged. The reason for her weakness must be established.

The chronic degeneration of Madeline's body is taking its toll. "What's next?! This is wrong, they fix it. Then this is wrong and then when they fix that, well by then I've got something else. Is there no end to this?" There is a sense of pleading in Madeline's voice. She experiences loss after loss, her sense of self eroding as each new symptom surfaces.

Despite the onslaught of new symptoms, despite all that is happening to her, Madeline remains hopeful. She describes herself as being in an immense hole; swallowed by something larger than herself. Madeline will climb out, however, as she has over the past eight years.

I'm sure we'll get through this and we'll look back and I'll think, "Well, it couldn't have been that bad." It's just like when you're in it and feeling miserable and terrible that you just sort of feel that this hole is just getting deeper ... and how am I ever going to get out of here?

The neurologist detects no abnormalities. Madeline has pain without an explanation. Cancer pain as mystery. The results of the scans are also clear. Cancer is not hiding in any of the body parts imaged. Madeline is referred to an oncologist who specializes in pain control. Oral Demerol has "held" Madeline for several weeks, but she begins to vomit again, she can no longer tolerate the Demerol. "I stopped taking the Demerol because I started throwing up again. It just hit me — bang, all of a sudden." Madeline goes to her medicine cabinet and looks at the six different pain medications lined up on the shelf. She decides to take one of her previously prescribed analgesics and it provides her with some relief. "That did make a difference, but I still have pain."

As quickly and mysteriously as it appeared, the pain in Madeline's arm vanishes. Radiation treatments scheduled for her arm are cancelled. During the second week of October 1993 she is awakened by a biting pain in her leg. "I woke up at five in the morning with such terrible, terrible pain in my leg. The pain is jumping around and they wanted to attack it with the chemo instead of the radiation." Madeline's oncologist orders a new chemotherapy agent — adriamycin. Her wandering pain of unknown origin presents as an oncological enigma. While the pain wanders throughout her body, Madeline can hardly walk. The combination of chemotherapy and the concomitant use of nine medications induces vomiting. Madeline becomes overwhelmed by the volume of medications she must take.

Okay, I had the chemo and then they put me on the onacitron [Ondansetron] — which was the anti-nausea. And then Demerol and the prednisone.... I was on Tylenol. I was on some kind of a stomach liner that was supposed to prevent the prednisone from causing upset and then there was something else, some more stuff.... I can't even remember what it was. But it was a lot at one time. Oh, I was on Stemetil and I stopped taking that because I was just shaking.

Evidence of Corporeal Corruption

An MRI (magnetic resonance imaging) scan reveals that cancer has spread to Madeline's right shoulder, at last providing an explanation for the pain and weakness in her arm. The medical puzzle is solved; cancer has advanced in her body. Madeline's oncologist hopes to stop the spread of her cancer with adriamycin. Madeline last took adriamycin in 1985 and suffered the side effects of severe nausea and vomiting. Her physician reassures her that the dosage will be less than what she received in 1985. Adriamycin memories surface and Madeline is apprehensive.

Madeline is placed on the synthetic opiate methadone at the end of October after consulting the pain specialist. Although she is aware that the methadone will require some time to control her pain, she remains ambivalent about taking this drug. She experiences nausea, which she attributes to the methadone. "I haven't noticed that it's made any difference. I threw up yesterday and I threw up today so I don't know whether it's going to work." Madeline lacks faith in the methadone. She has no reason to believe that it will ease her burden, given that nothing else has worked so far.

Madeline is now housebound. Without energy, without strength, and in constant pain, she ventures out from her home only for medical appointments or to attend church. The walls press in on her.

Like you're miserable and you're horrible and like when I was so sick, you just don't make that effort, that contact. It's just too much. And you're having so much trouble just concentrating getting through what you're dealing with that nothing else just matters. I feel bad. I mean I haven't talked to her [friend] and I haven't talked to her [another friend] and I haven't talked to her [another friend]. I don't want them to think I'm ignoring them. But in the meantime they don't know how sick I've been.

Madeline is incarcerated by this disease and its treatment. Unable to maintain contact with her friends, some of them begin to fall away. Cancer consumes her social body. Madeline channels all her energy into attending church service. "I try to get out on Sunday morning, depending on how I feel when I get up. I don't have the energy to do a lot more than that."

The Death of Madeline's Mother

In the course of Madeline's struggles with cancer, in the first week of November, her mother, weakened by amyotrophic lateral sclerosis, dies in a small rural hospital in Manitoba, not far from where Madeline was born. Madeline's oldest sister, a nurse, was with her mother as she died.

It was just her time. She was so tired. She was just so tired. She couldn't even lift her arms or anything anymore. She had no strength at all. She said very little and most of the time she was drowsy. She wasn't eating. She wasn't drinking ... oh ... she looked so terrible in there [the hospital]. And yet she had no pain. At least we can be thankful for that.

Madeline is thankful that her mother died without pain. Madeline and her family prayed that the Lord would not permit her mother to suffer. He answered their prayers.

The Lord's power is just overwhelming. We prayed for so many things and so many of them were answered. We just can't get over that. I prayed that she would have a quiet spirit, that she wouldn't be restless and anxious and stuff and I mean she just lay there quietly and you know she had no pain and you know we prayed for that too — so that she wouldn't be tossing and turning and in agony and in pain and stuff and I mean it was just one thing after another. He answered this and He answered this and He answered this.

The power of prayer, and moreover the power of God, is reaffirmed in the death of Madeline's mother. It was time. She was so tired. Madeline too is tired, but it is not her time. The week of her mother's death and funeral is a blur. Madeline goes out to her parents' homestead, but has to return to the cancer clinic within 24 hours to receive chemotherapy. Cancer treatment does not pause for life nor death. Madeline's blood count is low, but she takes her chemotherapy. The next day she returns to the clinic and receives three units of blood. She overnights in the city and then returns to her mother's funeral. Madeline states that it was only through the prayers of her church family that she had the strength to carry on. "There was so many people praying for me, without those prayers I don't think I would have made it through that week. Knowing they're behind you — that makes a world of difference."

It was just so much in one week, you know, so much in one week. It was incredible. And then Saturday of course, we had to get rid of all Mom's things. Dad says, "I can't look at those clothes. Just get them out of here."

Madeline sorts through her mother's clothing. Each piece of clothing holds a scent, a memory. Madeline presses one of her mother's favourite dresses to her face and inhales deeply. Her mother is there. Her fragrance, briefly captured in the threads, releases memories. As Madeline breathes the scented memories, she carefully places the clothing in green garbage bags. The clothes will be distributed to the poor. Madeline's father walks in and out of the bedroom several times before the closet is completely emptied. He cannot participate and he cannot stay away. He and his wife would have celebrated their sixtieth wedding anniversary in December.

Madeline's mother saved her children's art; the cards they made for her. Little treasures protected for 40 years.

She had things that we made in school like when we were in grade 1 or 2. She had a whole box of things and she'd always save all her cards and there were things that we had made in school. It's hard, it's hard to get rid of some of that, to just throw it out. This person is gone now and to just throw all her stuff out.... I'm very sentimental so ... I would see things and oh, it would hurt me to throw them out, but what are you going to do?

In disposing of her mother's things, in gently placing her clothes in the garbage bags, Madeline must be reminded of her own mortality and her thin hold on life. Some day someone will place Madeline's things in plastic bags and remark on the children's treasures that she too has boxed away.

The Consumption of Madeline's Body

Chemotherapy causes Madeline's hair to fall out again. Electric clippers in hand, she shaves her head at the front and sides while her husband shears her crown. The hair loss does not bother Madeline. "It's comfortable. I would be eating and the hair would be falling in my food, and at night I'd breathe in the hair on my pillow. And I thought, this is ridiculous." Madeline purchases a wig, a toque, and a kerchief. "I'm ready."

The pain in Madeline's right arm resurfaces. She cannot move this arm. Her doctor changes the pain medicine from methadone to sublingual morphine. Methadone made her vomit. Given her experience with pain medication, Madeline is not confident that the morphine will work. She is sceptical and adopts a wait and see attitude. A week passes and Madeline is not nauseated. She is able to tolerate the sub-lingual morphine and she is thankful.

During the last week of November, Madeline's chemotherapy is halted because her blood counts are too low. The pain in Madeline's left leg becomes worse. She can barely walk. The physicians debate whether or not to X-ray the leg since an X-ray was taken less than six weeks before. They go ahead, and discover a fracture around the circumference of the femur; her thigh bone is cracked just below the hip joint. Madeline is admitted to the hospital for surgery and, under local anaesthesia, has three pins inserted to stabilize the fracture. The doctors and nurses are amazed that she has been able to walk on the leg. For the first time in almost two months, Madeline does not have pain in her left leg.

While her leg "settles," pitting edema swells her ankles. "My ankles are so swollen. They have been for a couple of days." Her doctors' fingers leave indentations in her putty-like flesh as fluid pools in her legs. The doctors think that chemotherapy may be damaging Madeline's heart. A heart scan is ordered; it will reveal any cardiac abnormalities.

Madeline is under siege. Cancer manifests its presence, and symptom by symptom it burrows throughout her body. Madeline tires of the constant assault. She is frustrated. She is tired. She asks plaintively and with lament, "When is it going to be nothing?"

This is enough already! You know, is it ever going to get easier again or is this it? You know, there are times when you really think, like man, how much more is going to fall into my lap? It restricts you. Your social life is basically on hold because you can't really go anywhere or do anything because you're either hurting too much or you don't feel good or whatever. And now with this ice and snow [winter] I can't go anywhere without somebody with me. There's no way I would attempt that because it's far too dangerous. Now the hip doesn't hurt, but now this arm is sore, like … when is it ever going to be nothing? Like when is it ever, this won't hurt, this won't hurt, the leg won't hurt, the pain will be gone. There's always something that still isn't right.

Earlier in her cancer experience there were periods of "wellness" when Madeline would be free of noxious symptoms, of the cancer demanding attention. Recently, something is always wrong with her body. There are no periods of reprieve. Nausea, vomiting, pain, fractures, weakness, hair loss, her heart — an unending litany of physical misery.

Despite her faith, despite her trust in God, it is all becoming too much for Madeline.

*

Madeline died during the winter of 1994.

*

Whatever comes, the Lord's with me. And I think that's why I'm not worried about the future. You know, whatever comes, He will be there with me and when my time is over, well that's fine. I know where I'm going. I don't have to worry about that either and I can take one day at a time and enjoy it. Take whatever comes and make the best of it. That's about all you can do. My strength comes from the Lord and day by day He gives me what I need.

— Madeline, September 3, 1993

LESSONS LEARNED: MADELINE'S GIFTS TO US

Madeline's lessons are those of a woman who lived for almost a decade with breast cancer. A year or so before her diagnosis, Madeline had a premonition that she was destined for breast cancer. She feared cancer and her intuition led her to be uneasy. Although many people would readily dismiss Madeline's intuitive sense about her destiny with cancer, she was able to "see" cancer in her life. She felt that she had to be vigilant with this disease. Not all things in the universe are open to scientific explanations. Regardless of the label we might place on Madeline's cancer vision, it is important to acknowledge and act on our feelings about our bodies and ourselves.

Knowing Your Body

Madeline experienced pain in her right breast for several years. Her intuition and fear of cancer, combined with the pain in her breast, led her to consult her family physician. Her physician repeatedly dismissed her symptoms. At one time he stated, "It is nothing and at 33 you are too young to be at risk for breast cancer." Madeline faithfully returned to her physician and was reassured time and again that nothing was wrong.

◆ Trust your intuition and knowledge about your body. No one knows more about your body than you. If you believe that your body is telling you that something is wrong, then act on this message. Should your physician dismiss your observations and concerns, and you feel that something is wrong with your body, consult another physician.

◆ Unfortunately, people sometimes have to be persistent to obtain the health care they need. Persistence, however, can save your life.

◆ Although some cancers occur primarily in older adults, never accept "age" as protection from receiving a cancer diagnosis. Cancer can occur at any age — among the young or old.

In retrospect, in light of what happened to her, Madeline's cancer might have been discovered sooner had she sought a second opinion.

◆ Living with cancer requires courage, determination, and the support of family and friends. You may need to call on these resources throughout the duration of your cancer journey.

People with cancer may have to be assertive and make health care providers listen to them. This often requires courage and dogged determination.

Responses to Chemotherapy

Madeline responded violently to her chemotherapy. She did not know what the side effects were and what was considered "normal." Had she realized that her incessant vomiting and the loss of several kilograms in five days was excessive, she could have sought assistance at the cancer clinic. Madeline also experienced profound fatigue. This bothered her greatly as she was a person who prided herself in having limitless energy.

◆ Side effects vary depending on the chemotherapy used and from person to person. Although there are general responses to cancer drugs, what you may experience also depends on your body.

◆ Always ask your physician and the cancer clinic nurses what side effects are most commonly associated with the treatment you are receiving. Will your treatments cause weight changes, loss of appetite, nausea, bruising or bleeding episodes? Moreover, find out what can be done to reduce or manage these side effects.

◆ Have your health care providers explain the differences between a reasonable response and a severe response to chemotherapy.

◆ Hair loss (from your head, your underarm, and pubic areas) as a consequence of chemotherapy is temporary and usually occurs ten days to three weeks after treatment begins. The hair usually grows back after the treatments are completed.

◆ Some people gradually lose their hair while others literally lose it overnight. You may wish to purchase a wig (or rent one), baseball caps, scarves, or other head coverings before your hair thins or falls out.

◆ Some women and men do not hide their hair loss with a hat or head covering. They accept hair loss as part of their cancer experience. They also find wigs and other head pieces uncomfortable.

◆ Chemotherapy can cause a loss of appetite. Find out what you can do to stimulate your desire to eat. For example, some people take a short walk before meals or they eat small, frequent meals (five or six a day). Make sure you keep track of your weight. Report any weight gains or weight losses to your health care providers.

◆ Diarrhea can occur while taking chemotherapy. Limit high-fibre foods and foods that are greasy or spicy. Alcohol, tobacco, and caffeine can make diarrhea worse. Drink plenty of water every day (at least 3 to 4 litres) while you are having treatments.

◆ Nausea and vomiting: Ask your physician or your cancer nurse about antiemetic medication (to prevent or stop nausea and vomiting). Sometimes you will need to routinely take this medication while receiving chemotherapy. If you can't keep anything down, take clear fluids (such as water or apple juice) and call the cancer clinic for advice and treatment.

- Fatigue is a common response to chemotherapy. Try to conserve your energy as much as possible and plan for rest periods.

- Sometimes anaemia, chronic pain, depression, poor diet, and a lack of rest can contribute to fatigue. Your physician will regularly test your blood to ensure that your blood is strong enough to continue with chemotherapy treatments.

- If your blood reveals that it has been greatly affected by the chemotherapy, your treatment may be reduced, stopped, or changed until your blood volume returns to normal.

Madeline assumed that her responses to treatment were ordinary. Asking questions about your cancer treatment is important and can protect you from harm. Find out what you should expect given your treatment.

Keeping Life as Normal as Possible

Madeline wanted her life to be as normal as possible while she lived with cancer. To this end, she underwent breast reconstruction after her mastectomy. She wanted to look normal. Madeline was not pleased with the results of her plastic surgery. Her reconstructed breast was much smaller than she anticipated. She then underwent breast reduction of her left breast and she was still not satisfied with the outcome.

- Discuss your options regarding breast reconstructive surgery with your physician. If possible, ask your physician for the name of a patient who would be willing to talk with you about her experience with reconstructive surgery.

- A picture is worth a thousand words. Ask your physician if he or she has photographs of patients before and after their reconstructive surgeries.

- The loss of a breast can be devastating to a woman's self-image, self-esteem, and sense of sexuality. Reconstructive breast surgery may help you feel better about the profound changes to your body.

◆ Women may also decide not to have reconstructive surgery of any kind. Undergoing reconstructive surgery is a personal decision.

◆ Some people may experience sexual difficulties during and after treatment for cancer. You can talk to your health care provider about these things.

◆ Couples sometimes seek counselling to help them with the consequences of treatment. It is important to keep the lines of communication open with your partner. Talk about how you are feeling and what is happening to you. Talk with your partner about how he or she is feeling. Talk about your relationship.

◆ For many people who are living with cancer, life can never again be "normal," but they try to reclaim dimensions of their pre-diagnosis lives.

◆ Integrating cancer into the fabric of one's life helps many people to prevent cancer from dominating their lives.

In addition to reclaiming her body from the consequences of surgery, Madeline tried to maintain normal routines and processes. For example, she attended church, and regularly visited friends.

Spirituality and Cancer

Madeline's profound faith helped her to live with cancer. Her belief in God and her love of God made her cancer experience survivable. Not all people are religious, but all of us are spiritual beings. Spirituality exists in many forms. We can express and experience spirituality in many ways. For some people, organized religions such as Christianity, Judaism, Hinduism, Buddhism, and Islam provide spiritual nurturance. One of the major functions of religion is to "feed the soul" and provide comfort to those who suffer. For people who do not embrace religion, the arts including poetry, music, painting, sculpture, and drama, can help us as we struggle and suffer with a life-threatening disease.

◆ Expressing and nurturing your spirituality can help you in your journey with cancer.

◆ You may wish to talk with your rabbi, priest, pastor, or spiritual director about your cancer. He or she may offer you comfort in a way that your health care team cannot. Make use of the support available to you from your spiritual family.

♦ The arts can be a source of comfort for people living with cancer. Many of the great works in music, art, and theatre deal with the topic of human suffering. These pieces move our spirit and help us understand the human condition, the suffering we all endure as part of living. We are afforded much insight and understanding about being human and struggling with adversity through the arts. Moreover, the arts can be a source of comfort and consolation to people living with cancer.

♦ Some people who have never previously had one take up a hobby or begin to express themselves after receiving a cancer diagnosis. They "find" a way of expressing themselves and capture what is happening to them through writing, painting, ceramics, needlepoint, woodworking, or photography. Acts of creation and the expression of "the self" can be sources of comfort as well as "balm" for the spirit.

Attending to our spiritual dimensions, knowing that we are part of something larger in the world, can help us live with cancer. Religion, art, and love can transport us from our immediate circumstances and relocate us beyond space and time. Madeline's faith in God enabled her to live fully during her cancer experience. She was comforted by her faith and by her beliefs.

Freedom from Cancer Pain

Madeline experienced uncontrolled pain. The pain medication she was taking could not keep her pain free. In excruciating pain, she sought relief at an emergency department of a major urban hospital on a Saturday night. Given the available personnel and time resources, she had to present to the emergency room physician nine years of living with cancer in 5 minutes. Madeline could not recall all the pain medications she had been prescribed over the past six months. The physicians were not experienced in chronic pain control or treating people who were suffering from advanced stage cancer.

♦ *Pain control is one of the most important dimensions of cancer care.* Having cancer does not automatically equate to having pain;

however, any pain that surfaces should be dealt with quickly and effectively. Any pain that you experience should be responded to with some type of pain therapy.

♦ Find out from your physicians and nurses about "after-hours" pain management. Request a phone number where you can seek assistance on the weekend, in the evening, or at night. Assistance should be available to you regardless of the time of day or night.

♦ Make sure you tell your physician or nurse if you are experiencing pain. Your pain cannot be controlled unless you tell someone about it.

♦ Your physicians or nurses may offer you pain medication or they may encourage you to try alternative pain management techniques such as deep breathing, talking with others, focusing on other things, and relaxation therapy.

♦ An increase in your stress levels can contribute to an increase in pain. Stress reduction techniques can help reduce the pain that may result from stress.

♦ Being fatigued can also contribute to pain. Ensure that you don't get too tired.

♦ There are many myths about pain control. You will not become addicted to the medication used to control pain related to your cancer. Taking pain medication early in your cancer experience will not make pain control more difficult later on. Do not feel that you must suffer with pain in order to save the strong medication that may be necessary should your cancer advance.

♦ One of the possible side effects of opioids (medication such as codeine, Percodan, Darvon, Dilaudid, Dolophine, and morphine) is constipation — which does not diminish over time. Talk with your physician or nurse about how to manage constipation. You may require stool softeners and medication to increase your bowel activity. You may also consider increasing your fibre, water intake, or activities as tolerated.

◆ Some people experience nausea and vomiting while taking narcotics (opioids). The intensity of nausea and vomiting varies from person to person and the type of opioid they take. Your physician may order around-the-clock management of this side effect by prescribing medication to control these symptoms.

◆ If you are in pain, *it is not your fault.* Nor is it your fault if you experience nausea or vomiting. It is the responsibility of your health care team to do everything possible to relieve your pain and control your nausea or vomiting. Never hesitate to report if you are having pain, or if the pain medication you are taking no longer effectively controls your pain.

Madeline needed a pain expert, someone knowledgeable about morphine, breakthrough pain, and bone pain. Her experience in the emergency department was terrible. Although Demerol provided her with immediate relief, Madeline's pain resurfaced within three hours of this injection. She could not get her prescription filled until Sunday morning. These new pills, ordered by the emergency room physician, made her nauseated and she could not take them. Madeline was in pain all day Sunday and went to the cancer clinic when it opened on Monday morning. On another occasion with uncontrolled pain, Madeline chose pain over returning to the emergency department for help. It is important to ask your physician about how to access after-hours care. Where can you go if you are experiencing a problem? Whom can you call? Will a cancer specialist — a nurse or physician — come to your home? These are important questions that people who are being treated for cancer should ask of their health care providers. It is also wise to always have a phone number of a physician you can call in case of a cancer emergency.

Letting Family and Friends Know How to be Helpful

Planning ahead can be difficult when you are a person living with cancer. Madeline observed that sometimes you feel "lousy" on the day of a planned outing or event. Friends and family need to know that people with cancer have their good and bad days. Sometimes Madeline had the energy to do the things she wanted, and on other occasions, she was without energy. For example, it took her a whole day to clean a shower stall in her bathroom. A decrease in energy may require reassessment of priorities. Madeline was unable to keep her home as clean as she would have liked to given her fatigue, nausea, and vomiting. Sometimes people with cancer must give themselves permission to "let go" of things to conserve energy. Letting go can be difficult. This is where family and friends can help. People often want to be of help to people with cancer, but they are at a loss about what to do. Friends and family can feel helpless and awkward.

- There is no magic formula about "what to do" or "how to act" with people who are diagnosed and treated for cancer. Family members and friends just need to be themselves. They will look to you for cues as to how they should behave or interact.

- Awkward or uncomfortable moments can occur among friends who visit you for the first time, but these episodes are usually brief and fleeting. A person living with cancer needs good and loving friends who do not permit awkward moments to interfere in the care and concern for another who has cancer.

- Friends may want to bring something to the home of someone who is living with cancer so as to not feel uncomfortable. When friends ask what they can do — let them know. Ask them to bring food, or a book or magazines for you to read.

With permission of the person living with cancer, a cleaning crew or cooking crew can be particularly helpful and greatly appreciated by those trying to survive cancer. The women in Madeline's church took her boxes of home cooked meals. Madeline was appreciative and thankful. She benefited from the gifts these women brought: their company and their meals. Running errands for people who are living with cancer can also be helpful. Madeline became housebound as her cancer migrated to her bones and her joints. She was unable to leave her home except to attend church on Sundays. She appreciated having someone get her postage stamps and other items she needed.

Life Unfolds Despite Cancer

Madeline shared with us that despite cancer, life goes on. As does death. During the course of Madeline's cancer, her mother died.

- Whether you withdraw or engage in life — *it will unfold around you.*

- Good things and bad things will continue to happen to you — despite having cancer. Cancer does not stop the world from going forward. Seizing those life-moments, especially those filled with joy and laughter, will permit you to live as fully as possible.

Cancer is not a talisman. It does not protect us from life, from the sorrows and hardships that accompany the joy and happiness found in living.

Madeline's gifts were many. She helped us to understand that we know our bodies better than anyone else, including health care providers. We need to listen to our bodies and trust in our corporeal knowing. Madeline responded violently to her chemotherapy treatments. As a consequence of journeying with Madeline, we now know how important it is to find out the side effects of treatments. We need to know what we can expect and what we should report to our physicians and cancer nurses.

Keeping life as normal as possible was a great challenge for Madeline. She struggled to reclaim her body from the effects of cancer treatment. Moreover, she tried to maintain those routines and rituals that contributed to stability within her home. Madeline also tried to let her family and friends know how they could best help her as she journeyed with cancer.

Given that cancer can threaten our lives, we learned from Madeline that our spiritual selves can help us live with advanced cancer. How we express our spirituality does not matter. What is important is to "feed our souls." Madeline accomplished this through her faith, trust, and love in God, and through members of her church-family.

One of the most important lessons from Madeline concerns her experience with cancer pain. Madeline suffered because her cancer pain was not well controlled. The hallmark of good cancer care is satisfactory pain control. Madeline showed us what can happen when pain management is inadequate. Of all her experiences, this one was perhaps the most significant because of the great suffering Madeline endured as a consequence of her pain.

Finally, Madeline taught us that our lives unfold despite cancer, and that we will encounter all the joys and sorrows that life brings while living with cancer.

7

KAY

FAITH IN A CURE:
OVARIAN CANCER

KAY GUARDS HER ABDOMEN. Still recovering from surgery, she carefully rests her hands on her belly, protecting it from further assault. Her ovaries and uterus were removed less than a month ago. Both the operative site and Kay remain tender. She sits in her garden, surrounded by the purple hues of bearded iris and giant waxed begonias. This is Kay's space. Her place of comfort. Unlike the family members who encircle her, the flowers give of themselves and do not ask for much except water and the occasional gentle touch. Kay is a woman diagnosed and treated for ovarian cancer, a mother who comes to realize that her cancer cannot be controlled, that she will not survive this journey.

Long and lanky, Kay is visibly thin, but not anorexic. Wrinkles cascade down her face and pool at her throat. She looks older than 50. Angular and mannish in appearance, she often wears a plaid lumberjack shirt and jeans. Chopped by blunt scissors, Kay's blonde hair grows uneven and untamed from her scalp. Sapphire-blue eyes soften her coarse features. Kay's hands are big. Mechanic's hands. The hands, too large for Kay at this point in her life, reveal her history. At one time they held tire irons, chains, tow truck tools, and her marriage. Kay's hands now hold softer things; her granddaughter and flowers from her garden.

Kay has three children. The oldest, Roger, lives with her ex-husband in the country. The twins live with her. Matthew and Melinda are 18. Melinda recently had a baby, Erin, who is one month old. Like most teenagers, Kay's children are simultaneous sources of joy and heartache. Kay is close to her 84-year-old father. He phones her daily. When he visits, he is accompanied by Kay's stepmother. Kay unaffectionately calls her "the second wife."

Kay is responsible for many people. "All the time. My friends, my sisters, my children, my family." She looks after them, tends to them.

"I live for my family, everything's for my family." Rarely does anyone care for Kay. She generally rebukes offers of assistance, sympathy, or concern. Fiercely independent and proud, Kay can make it on her own.

And now my father is taking care of me *again*! Like I'm a baby. My girl-friends want to baby me. They want to take me away and baby me. My girlfriend says it's alright to cry. It's okay to let your guard down. I let my guard down just once cause she talks me into it and I just get emotional. The time isn't right yet. When the good Lord says it's time to come now … I'll say, "Okay now I can cry. I'll be there in a minute."

Kay does not want anyone to baby her, to treat her differently even though she has cancer. A self-proclaimed stoic, Kay permitted herself to cry once over cancer and she has come to regret it. Letting down her guard will come. This will happen when the Lord calls her. Kay takes no stock in the healing power of tears. "Cry for yourself, for what? It doesn't do you any good. It puts you on a downer." Beyond her iron will, Kay relies on God.

You can only ask God to help [you] survive this ordeal. No one else can help me. Like, my dad's there. But something, some greater strength has to come from above.

Kay looks to God for support, for strength, and ultimately for sur-vival. She is a spiritual woman. She prays God will take away her pain.

I asked Him to take the pain away. And He did. Because I just can't stand the pain. It just kills me … it just defeats me. So He's eased up on the pain.

God hears her prayers and eases her pain. Her faith is great.

It is faith that gives you the strength to get up and say, "Today I'm going to do something different." It has to come from God. He has to just … help you.

Kay, her twin children, and her grandchild Erin live in a tiny wartime home. Green and white, it looks like a child's playhouse. They live in the north end, the poorer part of the city where Kay survives on social assistance. From her backyard, from the vantage point of her garden, a funeral home is visible: Jorfe's. Kay sits with her back to the funeral home. She refuses to face it.

The Early Years

Kay was born in a small Manitoba town called Stoney Plain. She states she was "delivered on a rock pile." Stones. Kay is destined for a hard life. "I should have been a boy." Her father really wanted a male child, and he got Kay and two other daughters. Kay is the oldest. Despite her gender, her father treated her as a son and taught her about machines, engines, cars, and trucks. She became an accomplished mechanic as an adolescent. Kay's mother often yelled, "She's a girl!" in attempts to reclaim Kay's feminine side.

Life in Stoney Plain was spartan. Kay describes her family life as simple and her parents as religious people.

It's simple. You work, you get fed, clothed, you go to church on Sundays. Sunday school in the morning, church at night and sit around on Sunday. You can't do anything. Just sit. "Oh you're not doing anything today, this is Sunday." No cards.

Hers was a no-nonsense Presbyterian family. "We were brought up almost like Catholics." No makeup, no smoking, and an assortment of rules and regulations. Kay's mother told her that she would get pregnant if a boy touched her. "A fellow put his arm around me and I waited for nine months to see. I thought, 'what a liar, she's a little liar.'" Discipline was physical. "Father could hardly get in the door without mother saying, 'Oh they were bad today,' and he'd give us a smack."

At 16, Kay's mother forced her to leave home — a ritual to be carried out with all the daughters. Her father opposed the move. Kay left home and worked as a sales clerk at The Hudson Bay Company for 13 years. One of her best customers was her ex-husband Dale. He would purchase inexpensive items, small costs for the pleasure of having Kay wait on him. She became pregnant, married, and helped her husband start a tow truck business. The marriage was a disaster, lasting only three years. Dale's extramarital affair, his thieving, and his physical abuse of Kay ended the marriage.

Cancer in the Family

Cancer is familiar to Kay. Anyone she knows with a diagnosis of cancer has died, including her mother-in-law, Ruth.

The cancer clinic asked, "Are you familiar with cancer?" Oh yeah, I'm familiar alright. My mother-in-law had it, died from it. And anyone I know.

Kay recalls Ruth's experience with cancer. Witnessing the cancer ravages endured by her mother-in-law was painful for Kay.

Well here's a slap in the face. She had it in the same area as me. Never had herself checked and her death wish was that I would have myself checked every year. And it scared me when she got it because she was in her fifties and too young to go. And I had an old nurse next door to me that said, "Stress is the worst thing for cancer." And that's exactly what my husband gave my mother-in-law. That's what I seem to have here ... is a lot of stress. I find it seems to upset it [her cancer]. But my mother-in-law had cobalt, chemo, she really went through the mill with it. All I wanted was for it to stop. She went from about 185 pounds to maybe 70. And I thought, God! Maybe that's what scares me when I look in the mirror.

Weight loss, hair loss, and the loss of self. Frightening, foreboding memories of her mother-in-law's earlier dying. Looking in the mirror frightens Kay. It is as if the mirror is a "looking glass" to the future in which Kay sees her mother-in-law's face staring back at her; a cancer visage.

The Later Years: Diagnosis of Bilateral Ovarian Cancer

Kay describes the symptoms that brought her into contact with the health care system. Her belly swells. It blossoms as it did with her first pregnancy. What is held in Kay's belly cannot be birthed.

I noticed it on Mother's Day. I blossomed out like a nine-month pregnant woman, in three days. I went up to 170 pounds from 150 and my pants kept on expanding about two inches every day till Wednesday. From Monday to Wednesday and then I was full bloom like a nine-month woman's pregnancy.

Kay notices gross changes in her body on Mother's Day. A grim coincidence. Her body reproduces, but not a fetus. The very organs that have contributed to life become harbingers of death. Kay will once again labour, this time for her own life.

I phoned HouseDoc [physician home visiting service] and one doctor told
me it was gas … he gave me gas pills. I took those till Saturday morning.
I phoned again and a young fellow came in and he said, "You've got a block-
age of some kind. Go to the hospital and get it examined." They wouldn't
touch me at the hospital until they got a urine sample because they thought
I was pregnant.

Wanting to rule out pregnancy, the physicians request a urine sample from Kay. She is not pregnant. "But as soon as they got the urine
sample, then they got scared." The young physicians in the emergency
department sense something is terribly wrong. It is serious. They
become alarmed, frightened. The doctors-in-training ask Kay if she
was aware that something was wrong before Mother's Day. Kay recalls
knowing something was there six months before her belly mimicked
pregnancy. In December 1992, Kay had experienced pain in her
abdomen.

Those little machete guys were in there and I could just feel them. And I
thought, "What is that sensation around my navel?" It was just, just like I
say, just like somebody was, with a little knife, or sword, just cutting away
in there.

Machetes in her belly. Stolid, Kay did not attend to her discomfort,
to the swords slicing through her abdomen. She seeks medical care only
when her symptoms become unbearable—some six months later. "The
surgeons, they helped me. 'This will be cleared up with the knife' and
boy it was." The surgeons excised a mass from Kay's body, along with
all of her reproductive organs. They also drained three litres of fluid
from her abdomen. This provided Kay with immediate relief.
But the surgeons, exact with their knife, are less precise with their
words. Telling a woman that she has advanced ovarian cancer is much
more difficult than removing cancerous organs from a body.

Well they didn't seem to want to say the dirty word. They just say, "Well,
we're talking the big one here now"-type of thing. I mean, you darn well
know when they say "the big one," we're talking cancer.

Euphemisms soften the blow. Gentle language for a cruel disease.
"They" cannot say the dirty word. It's too difficult for them to tell Kay,
even though this is about her life and death.

Kay is diagnosed with bilateral ovarian cancer. She is tough. Her father taught her to always be in control of her emotions, and she does not cry. Her girlfriends would have cried. Kay handles whatever comes her way. She confines her emotions to her heart.

Kay's Beliefs about Cancer

Kay believes that cancer is a sexually transmitted disease and she has brought this disease upon herself. By straying from a chaste life and enjoying the sexual company of men, she thinks that she brought this cancer upon herself.

I think what I've got is a sexually transmitted disease. Yeah, because I can't figure it out any other way. I tried to doctor myself for quite a few months and ended up going to the doctor and she gave me four pills [possible treatment for a specific sexually transmitted disease] and I took them just like that. The druggist gave me some for my friend and I said he could buy his own. I'm going down to tell him the good news, that he's got something and he doesn't even know he's got it. And my doctor never even checked me. She never opened me up. ... I was so raw from trying to treat myself. I thought I could take it away with vinegar and baking soda.

Vinegar and baking soda vaginal douches. Kay tries to treat what she thinks is a vaginal infection for several months. The self-treatments excoriate her skin and burn her raw. When these treatments fail to cure her, Kay consults a family physician who then prescribes her medication without any examination. Kay believes the cancer took hold during the time she tried to treat herself. Cancer as a sin of the flesh. It is a punishment of some kind for Kay's encounter with her male friend six years ago. Her last dalliance.

The Will to Live and the Treatment of Cancer

One week after her surgery, Kay commences chemotherapy. Initially, she thought she would refuse the chemo treatments. "I had always said, 'I'm not having chemo ... if I get cancer, I'll just die, I'll just let it eat me up and I'll just die.'" Kay changes her mind about the chemotherapy.

It seems once you get cancer, or once you know you have it [voice quavers] then you say, "Hey, maybe I want to save my life" [starts to cry].

Kay is scheduled to receive nine courses of chemotherapy. She refers to chemotherapy as "rat poison." It gives her body an air of chemicals, a heavy-metal kind of smell. "I can smell it. It seems to come out of my body or something." Infused through her veins, the chemotherapy surfaces on Kay's skin and permeates her life.

Yeah, I get a whiff of it and I think, "Oh God. I can't stand the smell." You know, that's the chemo and I think that's why I don't stay overnight in the hospital [after receiving chemo] because I can smell it there.

Chemotherapy must save her. She must live. Her children need her, they need their mother. They are Kay's reason for living.

And I put a lot of pressure on the doctors because I said, "I have three kids I have to [sobbing] take care of." [ten second pause] You know, and it's uh, that's what I think when it comes down to it ... I can remember my mother-in-law had cancer. She thought the same thing. She has to take care of the family. That's what made her keep hanging on and not give up. It's just the kids.

Kay cares for everybody, including her physicians. Tenderly, she states that she has placed tremendous pressure on them by seeking medical attention so late in her disease. Yet they must save her for the sake of her children. They cannot let her die. "I even asked them, 'Have you ever lost anybody?'" Kay wants reassurance. She wants a guarantee of survival.

They have to take on the responsibility of my kids with me. To make sure I could survive. They, they pulled me through surgery and now I sort of hate to give up on myself. I figure they can do anything. It's up to them now.

Treating cancer is an onerous responsibility. There is much at stake and expectations can be so unjust. Kay's cancer may be beyond the limits of her oncologists and the medical system. Kay, however, has faith in her physicians. She trusts them. They pulled her through her surgery. She cannot give up on herself, nor will she allow the physicians to give up on her. This is why Kay tells them about her children, why it is important for her to live. In her will to survive, Kay accords divine power to her principal oncologist.

And his eyes breathed life into mine. He had the most … penetrating eyes … almost like an ocean washing over me. I thought, "Oh my God. He, he's sent by God" … and I think that's why those guys are in there. I think [starts to cry] that they're God's right-hand men. And they know how to fix you up. And they know how to make you trust them. If I didn't trust them, oh man, I told them right from the start I wouldn't let them near me.

The physicians are doing God's work. God has sent them to save her, to "breathe life" into her. Eyes so powerful they breathe life into another. Ocean waves surge over Kay in the presence of this oncologist. She is cleansed; a kind of baptism occurs. She trusts her oncologists completely and entrusts them with her life. Baptized, Kay is now a believer in medicine. The physicians have the gift of healing and they will save her from her broken, diseased body.

The initial effects of chemotherapy become apparent. Kay's hair begins to fall out. A friend offers to trim it.

My girlfriend, she butchered my hair before I went in. She nursed her father when he was at the end with cancer and I thought, "Oh God. She knows something." And she's crying and she's bringing her daughter to see me. Like I'm at Jorfe's already. You know who the Jorfe's are? The funeral home. I thought, "Oh yeah, she knows something." She took my hair and chopped it off and I thought, "Yeah, I got cancer alright." Yeah, big time now. Hair's gonna fall out and everything. I brush it and I get a good brush full of hair every time I brush it. But she keeps on saying, "It'll grow in nice. It'll grow in nice." Yeah, my mother-in-law said that too. If I live long enough, my hair will grow in nice.

"Butchered" is how Kay describes her hair now. It is a marker, a sign that Kay is a cancer patient. Her mother-in-law was a cancer patient; her hair did not have a chance to grow in before she died. Despite her friend's reassurances, Kay recognizes that, for her hair to grow in "nice," she must live long enough. The fast-growing cancer claiming her body and the slow-growing hair highlight the jeopardy of a person with cancer.

Kay thinks she feels the little swords starting up again. She is not certain whether this is her imagination or the cancer is actually stirring inside her. What is real and what is imagined blur.

I wonder if what I feel in my stomach. I have to ask him [the oncologist] next time I go … the little swords that I felt before … do I imagine I feel them again? Cause sometimes I don't know if it's … my imagination or if it's just … starting up again.

Kay can handle just about anything. "But this damn thing I can't. This cancer just scares me to death." What frightens her is the possibility of her cancer returning and claiming her life.

That it's gonna start up again. That the doctors are not going to get it arrested. That they're just buying me time. I don't, I don't want to be bought time. I want, I want life. I'm greedy. I want as many years as my father if not more. I mean I haven't lived yet. [crying] I have my family. And now when I'm going to have my next 50 years, and now they're gonna take that away from me. [crying]

Kay wants her cancer arrested, incarcerated, locked away. She fears that she might be living on borrowed time. What she wants is life — nothing more, nothing less. Cancer robs. It too is greedy.

Existing — Between the Land of the Living and the Dead

Kay speaks of existing and not of living. "Either you're living or you're not. What's this existing?" The ovarian cancer path situates Kay between the living and the dead, moves Kay back and forth between these two worlds. At times she feels closer to the dead: "This past week I felt like committing euthanasia." Fatigue immobilizes Kay and makes her feel like she is dying. Other times, after the side effects of her chemotherapy have subsided, she embraces the living. "For the next three weeks I'm going to be full steam ahead. Then I go back for chemo again." This is the dance of chemotherapy.

Sometimes Kay cannot believe that she has cancer; that it has consumed so much of her life. "I look in the mirror and I think, 'Oh God! Why can't somebody else be there?'" Could someone else not take her place? It is the timeless plea of those who face suffering.

Melinda, Kay's daughter, gives birth to Erin in June 1993. The baby brings much needed joy for Kay. As with all newborns, Erin requires much attention and Kay frequently does not have the energy to look after her. This reinforces Kay's state of existing.

I should be up washing her bottles for her and getting things, getting the formula ready for her. I should be able to say to her [Melinda], "Just stay

in bed and have a good rest and recuperate. And I'll take care of the baby."
But I can't.

Being a grandmother is hard work. Kay cannot look after the baby
as she desires. Cancer, chemotherapy, and pain restrict her abilities to
give of herself. The baby develops colic. Melinda begins to shirk her
parenting responsibilities. She is much too young to be straddled with
motherhood and Kay is much too sick. Kay tries to pick up where
Melinda leaves off, but she is tired.

The first week with chemo and just everything — the baby, my daughter,
everything seems to be coming to a head. When I'm with the baby or my
son's with her, everything's quiet. She sleeps you know. But when my
daughter's home, she's constantly fussing. And her piercing screech. My
daughter gets fed up with the baby and she wants to go out.... I said to her,
"I can't take it day and night you know." She wants to go out in the night
time. It's too much!

Things become difficult and Melinda and Erin move out at the end
of August. It is all too much for Kay. The cancer, the chemotherapy,
her daughter, and the baby.

Kay as Innocent

In July, Kay notices a lump in her left groin area. Except for its presence, it does not bother her. By the end of August the lump has grown
to the size of an egg. It is visible through her jeans when she sits. The
physicians are concerned about this growth. They mention radiation
and this takes Kay by surprise. "So the doctor started keeping an eye on
it. He figures the chemo will arrest it, but, if not, then he said radiation. And I said no." Radiation frightens Kay. She has seen it burn the
people she loved.

Well, my mother-in-law didn't like it and then my aunt's niece up the coast
had a rare disease, had a rare cancer. And they burned her raw. They gave her
… 72 hours of it and the chemo too. This [tumour in her left groin] would
have to get awfully, awfully big for me to get scared of it and have to go in.

This egg-sized growth does not frighten Kay. She will accept radiation only if the lump becomes awfully big. "I figure it's just maybe an

inch and a half in radius." An ovoid lump appears in Kay's breast which she also considers small. Kay's point of reference is her body. These lumps are small when compared to her limbs and her torso. In reality they are significant serious metastases. "What's a little more cancer in you now that you've had 'the big one.'" Egg-like tumours incubate throughout Kay's body. Kay does not understand what these foreboding lumps are and what they mean. Innocently, she states "It's just a little piece of cancer here and there." Unlike the stabbing pains in her belly, these lumps are not painful and do not warrant Kay's attention. The lumps are just there.

Kay believes that her surgeon removed all the cancer and that the chemotherapy would kill any stray cancer cells. She is reassured by her surgeon's words, "After surgery you'll be 100 percent." It is a promise of great comfort. Kay remains encouraged by these words. "And except for these lumps I'm not too bad."

Ravages of Chemotherapy and Cancer

Chemotherapy poisons Kay's hair roots, they die, and she begins to lose her hair. Exasperated with her hair falling out in clumps, she takes her son's hair clippers and shaves her head. Matthew, her second oldest son, says to his mother, "It's not that bad old lady. It doesn't look that bad." To conceal her loss Kay wears a pink turban with someone else's blonde hair sewn into the material to create the illusion of luxuriant bangs. "I'm bald. I'm bald. I'm afraid to look in the mirror."

The waistband of Kay's pants strains uncomfortably once more against her bloating abdomen. Kay accommodates the pressure by keeping her pants unfastened. Oddly, as her girth expands, she becomes gaunt. Cancer takes what it needs to survive at the expense of Kay's body. People start to notice how thin she is becoming. "I'm so skinny and I have no rear end now. My back is just straight." Kay describes going in for a physical examination.

They put a pad on the bed yesterday and I said, "Oh they think I'm going to wet it or something." The nurse said, "Oh, no, I just thought it might be a little bit hard on you." So she already noticed that I was skinny too.

The ravages and losses brought by her cancer make everyday things "a little hard" for Kay. In addition to body losses, there are losses of the self. Layer by layer, Kay begins to disappear. A migration occurs. It is a drawing inward.

This life is a worthless trip so I guess I'll be coming back again eh? Oh boy.
I was thinking the other day, "Gee I can't do anything now." I can't even
carry a baby anymore. I can't carry a baby, I can't do anything anymore.
I think, "Boy you're really good for nothing now."

Kay cannot carry a baby. And she has carried so many children in
her life. Lifting and carrying any weight causes pain in her abdomen.
"I've always lifted heavy stuff all my life. Ever since I carried a pail of
water. Two pails of water — I could swing them around over my head
and not spill a drop out." Unable to carry even an infant, Kay feels she
is of no use.

There is much family tension now. Kay does not have the patience
she once had. Another loss. No one seems concerned about her welfare.
Her children want money, they want food and, like her cancer, they
always seem to want to take from Kay.

Well I jumped down the elder one's [oldest son] throat and then I proceed-
ed to follow down the other, Matthew's, throat. My older one said, "What's
with your attitude?" I said, "I don't know. Do you need money? What are
you here for?" He said, "No. I don't need money." Melinda comes in here,
waltzes in, says, "The baby's in the car and you can go out and look at her if
you want. Can I have some money?" Not, How are you? How are you feeling? Just money, money, money, or food or whatever you have. The oldest
asked me if I was scared. Who the heck can be scared? You haven't got time
to be scared. You're so busy worrying about where your next dollar is
coming from.

Kay gives much of herself to her children, but the cancer is taking
much of what Kay has to offer. There is very little left for her to share
with her family. Her eldest son knows that something is terribly wrong
with his mother. He asks if she is frightened. Kay replies that she is not
scared. Living on welfare means worrying about money and not other
things — like cancer. Beyond her financial concerns, Kay is fearful.
She hesitates to acknowledge the fluid accumulating in her belly. Her
enlarging belly means that the chemotherapy is not working. Kay
cannot consider this possibility.

My nurse friend says, "What are you holding your stomach for? Is the
chemo not working?" And that scares me because chemo arrests that fluid.
I think it's just that I hurt.

Kay holds on to herself for life. The physicians order a barium enema to rule out the spread of cancer to the bowel. They reassure Kay that the procedure is routine. "They like to know everything about me." Kay does not tolerate the procedure well.

My goodness, they know everything now. Turn this way, turn that way …
and this young fellow there saying, "It's alright, it's alright," and I'm crying,
for the first time I'm friggin' crying in there … and I thought, "It's just as well
that I'm going through this punishment right now and gettin' it over with."

From Kay's perspective, the test is punishment. Unjust sentences are associated with having cancer and, for Kay, the barium enema is one of them. She cries. "I'm friggin' crying in there." While Kay takes pride in being able to handle almost anything, this is too much. The test assaults her. It turns her insides out. They are on display, viewed on the television monitor. At the conclusion of the test, the technician says, "Now that wasn't bad, was it!" Her ordeal diminished and dismissed, Kay wonders aloud to the technician, "How can you make your living torturing people like this?"

Chemotherapy treatments continue. Kay experiences nausea and diarrhea. She speaks of her chemotherapy as if it were a living creature. "I'm nauseous today. It doesn't seem to like jelly beans." Sweet things now sicken her. Changes in her palate make her favourite foods nauseating. Accompanying the nausea is the pain in her abdomen. "I get those knife-like stabbings in there. On either side." Kay holds herself tightly when speaking of these pains. She cradles her belly as if trying to keep the cancer contained inside her abdomen.

Toward the end of September, Kay begins to talk about death. For the first time during her journey, she is truly frightened.

I said I was scared [to a girlfriend] and she said, "Of what? That's the first
time you've ever said you were scared of anything." And I said, "I'm afraid
my hair's not going to grow back in again." I said, "Wouldn't it be terrible if
I don't live long enough for my hair to grow back in and then I'd be in my
coffin like this? Because my mother-in-law was." What we went through
with my mother-in-law, it hits me too.

Kay's mother-in-law died while taking chemotherapy, before her hair had a chance to grow back. Kay is taking chemotherapy. Her hair has fallen out. Familiar with her mother-in-law's cancer history, Kay fears death.

Feeling Better: A Reprieve

At the beginning of October, Kay experiences a burst of energy. Feeling better, she celebrates her movement toward recovery by cleaning the home of a girlfriend's mother. Forever giving of herself, the selfless mother, Kay cannot help but look after this woman's home.

I'm feeling better. I cleaned my girlfriend's mom's place the other day. I wanted to see if I could do it. I didn't get pooped out or anything. I made her bed, did her washing, made the bed back up again. Hung her clothes up, washed her floors, vacuumed and washed all the bathroom down and everything.

Kay is convinced of her healing. "I'm on my way to recovery. I went down and bought a wig." Once again, Kay begins to take an interest in her appearance. Until now she has worn a turban. Now she invests in a wig, in her future. It will make a difference in Kay's appearance. It will make her feel better about herself. Even the pain in her belly seems to have diminished. Kay attributes some of the residual pain to healing and some of it to strain. "Maybe I strained myself or something." The reprieve lasts one month.

A Narrative of Dying

November. Kay's situation becomes grave. With her head shaved and the skin growing taut over the bones of her face and hands, Kay looks like a prisoner of war. She walks with her head bowed. Her arms cross and carry a distended belly. Kay lists. The weight of cancer presses her down. She wears a pink down-filled parka. It grazes the road while she floats, spirit-like, along the asphalt. Padded, the parka wraps around her hard, bony body. The coat is one of the few soft things in her life.

The chemo is leaving her more and more tired, it does not seem to be working, and Kay hates it. Chemotherapy used to make her feel good after a time. Now it induces a continual heavy tiredness. She feels drained of energy. "Before when I used to get it, I used to be really raring to go. I could cut the grass and everything." That was two seasons ago, in the spring. The lump in her left groin has grown so "awfully, awfully big" that Kay permits herself to undergo radiation. The lump shrinks in size. Kay is relieved.

Then the pain in Kay's belly worsens. She speaks again of knives, daggers, and machetes.

Sometimes it cuts me like a knife. My son has prayed to take some of the pain, too, because when I got my pain last night, he got his too. And I said, "Don't ever wish my pain on you. Just let me handle it. I can handle it." He gets it around his heart. So whether it's a sympathetic pain, maybe it's fright.

Matthew prays to ease his mother's burden and to share her pain. As Kay is gripped by the pain in her abdomen, Matthew suffers pain around his heart. It may be sympathetic pain or the pain of fright. It may also be the pain of a heart breaking. Kay refuses to allow her son to take some of her pain. She tries to feel better. She wants to be better. "I just want to, I want to get better." But she knows that her circumstances are not good, that she may be dying.

I'm feeling the pits. The pain's terrible. I don't know. I don't know why it doesn't get better. I try not to think of everything that I have to do ... get my house in order ... just in case it happens. [15 second pause] My back's so sore. I can't put on, how come I can't put any meat on me? I try and try, my gosh, everything I look at I eat. Constantly eating. Oh gosh, this is getting worse.

Significant changes occur in Kay's living habits. She can no longer eat a whole meal in one sitting. Like a sparrow, she flits back and forth from the kitchen table to her bedroom. It takes all her energy just to eat a little food. She must lie down and rest frequently.

I ate my breakfast and I ate my dinner in two parts. I eat a little bit and then I go and lie down and then I get up and I eat a little bit more and then I go and lie down. I'll do the dishes and then I'll go and lie down and get up and make my bed and then go and lie down and then do something else. And my neighbour says, "Don't tire yourself out." I said, "How can I? I have to have a rest after every darn thing I do." I go to the laundromat. I can't stay there because you have to sit down. I can't sit down unless I crouch down. And everybody is wondering "what the heck is she doing down there all crouched over?"

Sleeping becomes difficult for Kay. She cannot get comfortable. Weight loss and her painful swollen belly prevent her from sleeping well.

I can't lie on my tummy. I can't lie on my side and it's so hard on the back ... all the time lying on your back. It got so sore, bedsores almost. I don't see anything there, but I sure can feel it.

A neighbour friend suggests that Kay obtain a sheepskin pad from the hospital. The thick lamb's wool will provide some comfort. Kay's pelvis cuts through her paper thin skin. She needs protection from her own bones.

Kay mentions her grandchild and becomes animated. Arms embrace the air just as Kay does this child. The love of Erin is present in her voice, in her face. In the joy of the telling about Erin, there are tears of joy and sorrow in the same breath.

All you have to do is just touch her like that and she's giggling. Just the nicest smile and just laughing like a two-year-old. Like a little girl; a high giggle. Hangs on for dear life to everything. And I just put my head down and say, "Oh, you are so beautiful" and she's just laughing. She thinks everything's funny.

When she is with Erin, Kay's pain eases. Erin relieves what the pain medication cannot. The love for this beautiful child has narcotic properties. Erin heals Kay, if only for the moment. "She just makes you happy; the pain just goes away."

"God sent you, Erin, just to take that friggin' pain from me." I just, I don't have any pain when I'm playing with her or just enjoying her. [Kay is crying] Oh dear, I wish my daughter would bring her over more often, but she stays in too much.

It is now the end of November and Kay receives radiation to her lung; the ovarian cancer has spread to other parts of her body. Her oncologist changes the chemotherapy when Kay notices more lumps growing throughout her body. Masses appear at the top of her abdomen and in her right groin. "I don't know if I had one there before or not. I don't want to know anymore."

Changes occur in the demeanour of Kay's principal oncologist. He no longer jokes with her. He is serious, sad. Vanished is the power that Kay once ascribed to him. His eyes no longer penetrate, they do not wash over her.

He came in. They had sad faces. They didn't seem to be joking around. I thought maybe they lost somebody or something didn't work out. But I, I think then they know that they had to have, start this other radiation on me and so this time he came in and he just did the check and he said, "It's all in the lower area again … and we're going to try new chemo." And then he went around to the other side. I looked at the ceiling. And I said, "You're going to try the new chemo?" "Yeah" he says. And I said, "What if that doesn't work?" He said, "Well, we have to think positive." And I said, "And if that doesn't work?" And then he said, "Then there's nothing we can do." [10 second pause] I've been popping the Tylenol 3s, and praying the pain away. [10 second pause] I'm going to try the tea. I have to.

Kay's situation is serious. The oncologist does a check. He examines the body. Cancer has spread throughout Kay's lower abdomen. Her oncologist suggests they try another chemotherapy, something new, something different. Looking at the ceiling, perhaps toward heaven, Kay poses a courageous question. "And if that doesn't work?" Always instilling hope, the oncologist encourages Kay to be positive. As if reading his unspoken words, Kay pressures him again with her question. This time he makes a death proclamation: "Then there is nothing more that can be done." And it is in the silence following this pronouncement that Kay understands the terrible weight of these words. Her fate is sealed. Kay, born on rocks — who prides herself in her stoicism — cries.

I think Dr. X [oncologist] is awfully sad. He never even looked at me. I started to cry behind the curtain when he said there was nothing else after this chemo to try. He just turned and he was gone and I was behind the curtain and then I just walked. I never stopped for my yellow book [appointment book], nothing. I just went straight out. And that woman in the next bed to me, she's just happy as a lark and her hair is just getting so friggin' long. Look at mine!

Kay walks out of the cancer clinic. Her fate is carried in her body, her appointment book left behind. Kay, however, cannot flee her cancer. And the woman in the next bed is "Happy as a lark" with long and luxuriant hair. Kay, her scalp smooth, stumbles hard on her earthbound path.

Kay turns to God, to the comfort of her beliefs, praying that He will take her pain away. She will also try drinking an herbal tea which she believes will boost the immune system and fight her cancer. It is a matter of survival. "I'm going to try that tea. It isn't a cure, but it will give you some years, maybe. You never know."

Kay speaks of how difficult cancer is. The people who do not have cancer encourage her to "hang in there" and "not give in" and "to fight." Hopeful directives from the lips and the lives of the unafflicted. It is the canon by which people with cancer are instructed to live-and-die.

My landlady, she said, "Just keep eating. Just keep thinking positive. Just … don't give up, don't give in." So … but it's awfully hard when … like, you can't do anything. Like my girlfriend says, "It takes time." The minister said, "It takes time." You know, everything bad comes so fast and everything good takes so long.

Kay is tired. There are too many assaults to her body and her spirit. The assaults come quickly and much too fast to be offset by anything good that may happen to her.

The weight doesn't come on. I look in the mirror and I don't know who the heck is in there. And I can't work like I used to. [10 second pause] And I think that's what upsets me most. I don't want to do my afghans. I don't want to do my knitting. Nothing. Everything I try to do is ugly. I just have no, no design left. I think to myself, "What's God saving me for?" I haven't got anything left in me now. What's He keeping me here for? It's so hard.

Kay appeals to God to let her live, to spare her from the cancer, to just let her breathe.

I prayed to God, "Lift the burden from me. Just let me breathe. Let me live."

*

Kay died on December 31, 1994.

*

Matthew said he dreamt he was out decorating the tree, the Christmas tree out in the front yard and he said, "Your hair was that long!" [pointing to his shoulders]. I said, "I guess that's a couple of years down the road." I'll be glad when my hair grows.

— Kay, November 3, 1993

LESSONS LEARNED: KAY'S GIFTS TO US

Kay travelled a difficult path. She believed, hoped, and prayed that she would survive her ovarian cancer. Her will to survive arose from her children and grandchild. She could not die. These children needed their mother. Sadly, Kay did not survive her cancer. In her unyielding struggle with this disease, however, Kay offers us many lessons.

Accepting the Love and Care of Others

Cancer demands that we make changes in our lives. Some of these changes are easier than others. Kay could not relinquish her independence. Fiercely proud and emotionally conservative, Kay guarded her autonomy and self-reliance. Sometimes it is difficult to "let go" of those things that we hold dear in life, such as our desire to be as independent as possible. Enforcing our choices regarding these matters, however, may limit the expression of love in our lives.

- It is possible to maintain your independence and yet accept the kindness and care offered by others. You can set limitations and boundaries concerning what you permit to happen.

- Sometimes friends and family members need guidance in terms of how to be helpful or supportive. Let them know what you would appreciate from them and, just as important, what things you would not consider helpful. Suggest that they babysit, bake a casserole, take you out for a coffee or tea, or drive you to the cancer clinic — whatever would be most helpful for you is what people want to do.

- At times, during the course of your cancer journey, the words "I'm here" may be the most comforting words you will hear. Allow friends and family to be there for you.

- Some friends may be unable to cope with the possibility of your death and may disappear from your life.

- Most of your friends will want to be helpful and caring; however, they may be uncomfortable and unsure of how to accomplish this. Help your friends support you.

Kay generally refused those who wanted to help her and be of comfort to her. Friends and family often feel helpless in the face of cancer. Witnessing the suffering of someone we love leaves us feeling that we cannot do anything. We feel ineffective and unable to take action, although we desperately want to do something. Family members and friends may want to offer small acts of kindness to people living with cancer. These are sincere attempts to reach out to those who suffer from this disease.

Kay was a fiercely independent woman. She initially resisted overtures and offers of assistance from family and friends. Later, during the course of her cancer experience when she was seriously ill, Kay longed for the concern and compassion of others. It was at this point that she felt no one really cared about her or what was happening to her. No one recognized all the terrible things she was enduring. Even the oncologists to whom she entrusted her life eventually distanced themselves from her.

Tears for the Self: Emotional Cleansing

Kay identified herself as a stoic. She tried to keep her emotions "in check" and covered up at all times. Each of us has our own way of expressing our emotions. There is no right or wrong way to respond in situations involving our hearts.

- If you feel *angry — be angry*! Initially, you may just need to be *angry*. Then, after this initial expression, you may be able to engage in emotionally constructive expressions of anger. If possible, channel this energy into healing. Talk about your anger to those who will listen — yourself, others you trust, or members of a support group.

- If you feel *sad — be sad*! Shedding tears for the self will make you stronger, not weaker. Allow yourself some private time to experience your sorrow. Draw a warm, scented bath and play your favourite music and permit yourself tears of recognition for what is happening to you.

- Trying to maintain a false sense of "cheeriness" robs you of the opportunity to discuss your fears and anxieties. Maintaining any facade involves a great deal of emotional labour. You will need this energy for other things along the cancer path, like healing.

◆ Some people find that keeping a journal helps them to sort out what they are feeling while they journey with cancer. A journal offers you an opportunity to "voice" all of your emotions — to write them out and look at them as captured on paper. Looking at what you've written later in your cancer journey may prove helpful. You see your initial responses to cancer in a different light with the passage of time.

◆ It is normal to experience grief when you are diagnosed and treated for cancer. People lament and mourn the loss of their healthy bodies and lives. Some people living with cancer also develop depression. Signs that you may be depressed include persistently feeling down and finding that nothing you do lifts your spirits. Talk to your nurses and physicians about these feelings. You may benefit from a short-term course of anti-depression medication. You can also talk to family members, friends, or a counsellor.

Kay forced herself not to show what she was really feeling, and she berated herself when she did cry. Sometimes it is only in anger or sorrow that we validate the terrible things that are happening to us.

Listen to Your Body's Voice

Another aspect of Kay's stoicism concerned her health care seeking behaviours. Kay did not seek medical attention until she experienced considerable swelling in her belly. She ignored the sharp, stabbing pains in her abdomen for six months, until they became unbearable.

◆ Pain of any kind indicates a problem. It is your body's way of telling you that something is wrong. If you feel pain somewhere in your body, then seek out medical care.

◆ Very few cancers produce pain in their initial stages. The American and Canadian Cancer Societies can provide you with information about warning signs of cancer. As a person living with cancer, however, always pay attention to any pain you experience. Pain may indicate a change in your condition, the need to adjust the dosage or type of chemotherapy, or the need to initiate other kinds of treatment.

◆ Know your body well enough to detect any changes such as lumps or bumps. These lumps need not be painful to be cancer.

We need to listen to our bodies as they "talk" to us through signs and symptoms. Pain is but one voice our bodies use to command our attention. Kay's body spoke to her in other ways: increasing girth despite the loss of appetite, nausea, a lack of energy, the lumps in her groin, and constant fatigue. Sometimes, we do not "hear" what our bodies are tying to tell us because of all of the other "noise" in our lives. Kay, a single mother who was trying to survive on welfare had other things in her life that demanded attention. She suffered in silence for months until her symptoms — terrible pain and a swollen belly — finally moved her to action. Sometimes we do not hear what our bodies are saying to us because we may be frightened of what the message means. If you are frightened about a change in your body, talk to your health care provider about what you have discovered or observed.

The Need for Beauty

Cancer can rob us of much of the beauty in our lives. Surrounding ourselves with beautiful and comforting things can be restorative. They can help us heal. Kay's grandchild, Erin, provided her with much comfort. This child was an oasis of beauty in Kay's life. Holding Erin, just being with her was a great source of joy for Kay. The flowers in Kay's garden were another source of pleasure. Kay loved flowers. Her garden was full of her favourites — irises and giant begonias. Moreover, the garden offered Kay sanctuary.

◆ A place of refuge, a private space where thoughts can be collected and where reflection can take place is important for many people who are living with cancer. Retreating to such spaces can also offer opportunities for inner healing.

◆ A place of refuge may also be helpful to family members and friends.

◆ You may need to let people know where your place of refuge is or when you are going there — so people won't try to find you and intrude. Let others know when you need some time to yourself.

♦ Your place of refuge may include: a certain room in your home, a church, temple, or synagogue, a friend's place, a coffee shop, or a park. Your place of refuge may be a public or private space. You may want to be alone or you may wish to be a "stranger" among a group of anonymous people.

Joy and respite from cancer can also be found in everyday places, in familiar activities, and in relationships with those who love and care for us.

The Ebb and Flow of Cancer

Cancer is characterized by an ebb and flow of feeling "good" and feeling "bad." We need to take advantage of the periods of feeling good.

♦ Maximize your energy when feeling good. Do things such as connecting with new and old friends, visiting relatives, writing letters, or whatever else you determine as important.

♦ There is a difference between doing and overdoing. Listen to your body and "do" whatever does not cause you to be overly fatigued.

♦ These periods of reprieve, when you are strong and feeling like your "old self," are gifts in and of themselves — use them wisely.

Remember that your energy reserves are not limitless. During "down time" when your energy levels are low, rest is necessary. This is the time to focus on yourself and recover from the effects of chemotherapy or radiation. Always pace yourself and try to ensure that you do not overtax yourself.

Cancer as a Disease Affecting the Whole Family

Kay and her family experienced family tensions as her cancer progressed. Relationships within her family deteriorated. Overwhelmed with cancer and trying to survive, Kay began to lose patience with her children.

◆ Cancer not only affects you, but it also has an impact on all members of your family. Family members may become quite concerned about you. Talking openly about your cancer and your circumstances will provide family members the opportunity to process what is happening to you. Of course, some families do not "talk," yet much is said in this silence. You and your family have a pattern of communication that has been established over time. Remember that family members and friends may want to talk or reflect upon what is happening to you and them.

◆ Cancer will not make poor relationships better. In fact, the opposite is generally true. Existing family tensions will likely become worse. Some families require support in the form of counselling because family dynamics worsen with the arrival of cancer.

◆ Cancer affects every family differently. How it is handled is determined to a great extent by how the family has functioned in the past. If in times of past crises your family has pulled together and become closer, this may occur again. However, if previous tensions have fragmented the family, this pattern may again appear.

◆ Family routines often change with a diagnosis of cancer. Family members may need to "take over" jobs you once handled if you are weak, tired, or recovering from the effects of cancer treatment. Some family members may readily accept these new roles, but others may be upset. Try to keep the number of changes to a minimum. Sometimes it is a matter of adjusting a role, rather than dropping it. For example, you may have to prepare simpler meals and involve your partner or children in this activity.

◆ If family members cannot help each other, external emotional supports are available to the family. For example, there are support groups for family members. Check with your local Cancer Society or cancer clinic for information regarding support for family members. Find out what emotional supports are available to your family — and help them "connect" with these supports if appropriate.

- Children are bright and are capable of figuring things out. Trying to hide your cancer from them is not a good idea. You will want to talk with your children about your cancer and what is happening to you. Children can develop all kinds of fears — especially when their world is turned upside down and whispered conversations take place behind closed doors. Being open and honest with your children will enable them to understand what is happening to someone they love. If you cannot explain things to your children, consider entrusting this important task to a close family member or friend.

- Children will become aware of disruptions within the family. If you do not talk with your children about your cancer, then they will not know why bad things are happening within the family.

- Provide opportunities for your children to ask questions. Encourage them to tell you or a trusted friend how they are feeling.

- Children need reassurance, affection, guidance, and discipline at times of disruption in their routines.

- If there are family matters of great importance to you, make sure you take action, for example, legal direction, to ensure that things will unfold as you want them to should you not survive cancer. This will free your energy to focus on other things as you journey with cancer.

- All of us should have a will prepared — whether we are healthy or sick. Ensure that you have a will. You may also wish to establish a power of attorney, someone who will make decisions on your behalf should you no longer be able to do so. Some people have a "living will" made up. This legal document specifically instructs physicians as to your wishes should you become incapable of making decisions about your medical care. Check with your family lawyer or legal aid service regarding wills, living wills, and power of attorney.

Within Kay's family, tensions ran high and family members were quick to anger. Her children were trying to come to terms with their mother's worsening illness. Matthew experienced pain around his heart as Kay experienced pain in her abdomen. It was pain he felt for his mother and what was happening to her. Kay and her children might have benefited from counselling and support. A social worker might have assisted Kay to manage her financial situation. Family dynamics are always affected with the arrival of cancer and extra care must be directed to relationships and feelings within the family unit.

The Need for Excellent Pain Control

Kay prayed to God to take away her pain. She revealed the inadequacy of her pain management when she stated, "I just can't stand the pain. It kills me. It defeats me." Telling the physicians and nurses about her pain and obtaining effective pain medications may have provided Kay with relief from some of her physical suffering. Prayer is considered an effective behavioural intervention with low pain levels. Kay's pain, however, was severe and she required immediate relief.

- As a person living with cancer, your pain should be controlled at all times. Freedom from pain is the standard that members of the health care team strive to achieve. Let your nurses and physicians know immediately if you are experiencing any pain.

- *Do not suffer in silence.*

- Sometimes breakthrough pain occurs. This is a sudden, and sometimes brief, increase in pain even though you are taking pain medication. Your physician can order a "rescue dose" of pain medication over and above your regular pain medication.

Controlling cancer pain is critical to the quality of life experienced by people living with cancer. If you are in pain, consult your physician at the cancer clinic. Do not be afraid to be persistent in your efforts to obtain relief. If your oncologist cannot control your pain, then you may need a referral to a pain management physician.

Procedures and Tests: Asking Why

Kay's physicians ordered a barium enema to determine if cancer was present in her large bowel. Barium was instilled through her rectum into her large bowel. X-rays were then taken to "see" whether her cancer had spread into her intestines. This test was traumatic and it assaulted Kay. The barium enema was conducted in September and Kay died less than three months later.

- Find out what will happen to you during a "test." You need to know what will be done to you and your body. Don't just accept the name of a test. Ask what the test entails. Some tests are very uncomfortable and for some people unbearable. Know what you are getting into before the test is conducted. You also have the right to refuse any tests.

- The "story" you get from your family or friends about their experiences during a test may not be what you will experience. We are all unique individuals and their tests may have been done a long time ago.

- Do not be afraid to ask your physician why a certain test is needed. It is also important to ask what information the test will provide. How will this information *affect your treatment* — if at all?

- Ask your physician what it would mean *not* to carry out a particular test.

- Find out if less traumatic tests are possible.

- If a test causes you to suffer, let your physician know. Your physician may not know the specifics of your experience. Telling your physician of your experience with the test may help him or her better prepare other people for that test.

Asking about the purpose of a test and whether it is really necessary can be frightening, but living with cancer demands courage. Some physicians will not appreciate your questions. If you are not the kind of person who can ask questions of physicians, have a close friend accompany you to the cancer clinic. A close friend or family member can become your voice and ask questions on your behalf. Sometimes having someone with you can provide you with the courage you need to ask questions — or to challenge the need for certain procedures. Remember, this is your body, your life, and your experience with cancer. You are central to everything that happens and if you want it, you are entitled to have a say in what happens to you.

When Active Treatment Options End

For many people living with cancer, there comes a time when there are no more active treatment options. The disease no longer responds to chemotherapy or radiation or other forms of treatment. Some people appreciate the encouragement and hope offered by others at this point in their cancer journey: "Hang in there! Fight this! You can beat this!" Other people find these words demeaning given their circumstances.

- Many people begin to understand at some point in their cancer journey that they will not survive. If this happens to you, talk to your physician or nurse or spiritual director. Find out whether your intuition is correct.

- If your cancer can no longer be actively treated, find out from your physician what the plan of care will entail. How will the transition from active treatment to comfort care (palliative care) take place? What options and choices do you have at this point in your cancer journey?

- Remember that something *can always be done* about the symptoms you are experiencing, even if active treatment (for example, chemotherapy) is no longer effective. Your cancer journey does not end at this point. It continues, but requires a different medical approach to care.

- Some people choose to receive chemotherapy right up until a few days before they die. Other people stop chemotherapy and active treatments when they know that these treatments are no longer working to control the cancer or the symptoms they are experiencing.

- Ask your physician what hospital and community-based palliative care is available to you.

Friends and family members can be helpful and comforting by offering support that is appropriate to the person living with cancer.

Kay tried to be a good and loving mother. She did not always feel successful at this, given the ebb and flow of sickness caused by cancer. Kay's life circumstances, living on social assistance and single-handedly raising two teenagers and a grandchild, required almost all her energy. Caring for her family and trying to ensure their day-to-day survival consumed almost all her time and strength. Little of Kay was left for herself.

Accompanying Kay on her cancer path provided us with many lessons. She helped us to understand that cancer affects not only the person diagnosed, but every family member and friend. Each family member and friend journeys in their own way and at their own pace. Kay taught us the importance of accepting the love and care of others, and to have sympathy for the self. She also taught us that sometimes we listen to what our bodies are saying, but we cannot hear because of fear.

8

JOHN

A LONELY JOURNEY:
MALIGNANT MELANOMA

HEAVY-SET AND FLESHY, John's belly sags over his belt. His thick blonde hair is neatly barbered. His false teeth look inexpensive and too youthful for his face. Clean shaven, he wears wire-rim glasses, a thin beige sweater, and plaid pants. John places his right foot daintily on the ground with an unexpected nimbleness from this large man. Malignant melanoma took root in this foot. His left foot thuds heavily accepting his body weight. John's footsteps create a cancer cadence. Melanoma, the deadliest of all skin cancers, takes John on a cancer path of bodily consumption.

John is a smoker. Self-rolled, unfiltered cigarettes in the breast pocket of his shirt are his faithful companions. Cigarette smoke accompanies him and at times precedes his arrival in a room. Sprinkled with ash, his fingers yellowed, this habit marks John in the mingling of flesh and fire. John drinks daily, draft beer mostly. He is a regular at neighbourhood bars and at Royal Canadian Legions throughout the city's north end. It is not unusual for John to drink 12 draft beers a day. With or without alcohol, he loudly shares his ribald, earthy humour with anyone within hearing distance.

I had to go to physiotherapy and I used one of those, um um what do they call it, thrombolic [anti-thrombolitic] stocking. I don't wear it all the time. But I get a little fed up with it [laughter] once in a while. They're a pain in the ass to put on. You know for 45-50 years I've been trying to get into somebody's pantihose and now I'm wearing them. [Lots of laughter]

Acquaintances and drinking buddies surround John. Alcohol brings them together. He has few close friends.

John's manner is abrupt and gruff, confrontational, disruptive. These are the spoils of rule-bound systems he encounters. He pushes

systems to their limits and beyond. He issues ultimatums. When slight-
ed, John assumes a "To hell with you" attitude. This curt disposition
earns him a bad reputation among the cancer clinic nursing and medical staff. In these acts of resistance, however, John exerts what little control he has over what has become, for him, an uncontrollable cancer.

John lives by himself in a one-bedroom basement apartment. It
resembles an office. A large government-issue desk serves as his kitchen
table; a small filing cabinet, his coffee table. Surrounded by office arti-
facts, by mementos of a salesman's life, John sits in a wooden secretary
chair. The wheels permit him to spin effortlessly around his apartment
from his desk, to the coffee pot, to his computer station. An aroma of
strongly brewed coffee competes with the sour smell of single older
men who fend for themselves. John cannot sit still. He is always in
action; rolling cigarettes, making coffee, or cutting out grocery coupons
from the newspapers.

The Early Years

John was an only child born to Icelandic parents. His parents divorced
while he was a young boy. They sent him to live with his maternal
grandmother at Pelican Bay. Eight years later John's mother, Opal,
reclaimed him. Quitting school in Grade 10, he began working in a
bank as a teller. "I worked in the bank for a year and then I found out
how stupid I was and I went back and took my Grade 11. I graduated
and then I went out to work. I guess I could have gone to university or
something but it wasn't in the cards."

The Later Years

John is single. Married in 1959, divorced in 1980, he moved back to
Manitoba from Saskatchewan in 1989. He never remarried. Recalling
his "lady friends" raises a mischievous smile. John has four adult children: twin sons and two daughters. His children live in Saskatchewan,
away from John, creating the necessary distance between themselves
and their childhood memories of him. John and his oldest daughter
have not spoken for five years. Geography does not account for the
silence. Other more serious matters — distances of the heart — contribute to this troubled quiet. Abuse of his wife and children, alcohol,
and John's endless road trips led to his divorce and the emotional gulf
between himself and his children.

John's mother suffers from Alzheimer's Disease and he has placed her in a nursing home. This arrangement devastated John who was close to his mother. Her body is cared for in a small town near Winnipeg. Her mind resides elsewhere. When he visits, John takes her soft chocolate mints, jelly beans, and cigarettes.

We would go out for beers together and I would take her to the legion to play bingo. I would take her everywhere with me because her boyfriend passed away a number of years before and she never got involved with anybody else since then. So I would make sure she got out. I would make sure that she went to Vancouver every year. She had some friends out there. And I made sure she got to Saskatoon every two years to see the kids. The onset of Alzheimer's was completely frustrating. That just about killed me. To the point I was becoming a nervous wreck and having to get home care to come in and look after her and bathe her and this sort of thing. Because I just couldn't do it anymore myself. I put her in the nursing home.

Opal's diagnosis "just about killed" John. It robbed him of his mother and his best friend. Unable to provide the increasing hands-on care to Opal, John arranged the services of home care. Eventually she was admitted to a nursing home.

Cancer in the Family

John speaks about a daughter he fathered before he met and married his ex-wife. This daughter, Jan, is living with cancer at the same time her father is under treatment for melanoma. An odd twist of fate, but it is insufficient to bridge their distanced relationship. Neither Jan nor John re-establishes their disrupted connections with each other during their ordeals with cancer.

This is a daughter prior to me getting married. This is one I admit to but don't admit to. [laugh] And um, she lost all her hair. And she's what 35, 37, I guess. And um, she lived in Winnipeg here. And she's going through a real rough time. Um, she got hit by a truck in front of a dance club about two years ago and um … uh, broke her back, and she wasn't expected to walk again and she said bullshit, she's going to be riding her horses again. [uneasy laugh] And she fought it, but as a result of having the accident and doing all the CT-scans and everything, they found out she has cancer. So they removed her uterus and um, all the other stuff and she still had lots so she's undergoing chemo right now and she's just recovering from it.

John identifies with this daughter, but he cannot recall her age. He states that she is a fighter. Evidencing a strong, feisty spirit, this daughter is like John. "She said to hell with them and you've got to give her credit." To hell with them. John's creed. This doctrine will be repeatedly applied to the doctors and nurses at the cancer clinic as his cancer advances and its treatment falters.

John: Portrait of a Salesman

John has worked most of his life as a salesman. He is a salesman. It defines him and validates his existence.

I was the youngest restauranteur in Winnipeg. Um, in 1953 ... I belonged to the Canadian Restaurant Association then. That was fun. I was 18 I guess when I started my own restaurant out in St. Norbert ... and between my brother and myself, when we quit the restaurant and I started into selling office equipment and well, I sold Bibles first. And then I went into office equipment and pretty well stayed there for most of my life. But we had three restaurants, my brother and myself.

John continues to work as a salesman. He earns extra income through purchasing and selling surplus government furniture and office equipment while receiving a disability pension. It is an illicit activity. Earning this extra income makes him ineligible for the disability payments he receives.

Even though I'm on disability and that, um ... I try to do a few things. I've been doing a little bit of buying and selling from the government and um, um, and um I have a fairly large stall out at the flea market on Queen and Broadway right now that's probably two or three thousand square feet, full of office equipment, desks and chairs and filing cabinets and that, that I bought from the federal government and resold. So I'm in the process of doing that, however with the idea of chemotherapy now um it seems that to the point where I'm going to have to dispose of that stuff because um, if I'm going to be taking this treatment every couple of weeks [chemotherapy] I just won't have the energy for it.

Although John verbalizes that he needs to dispose of his inventory, his salesman's instincts override what his mind and body urge him to do. He does not sell off his stock. He cannot stop wheeling and dealing, making the sale. Every Saturday and Sunday he makes his way to his stall at a large indoor flea market. John sells desks, drafting tables, steno-chairs, dictating machines, cash registers, typewriters, computers, books, wall dividers, and filing cabinets. He purchases 25 room dividers from the Department of Indian and Northern Affairs. John will add these dividers to his inventory at the flea market. He cannot resist reselling merchandise. Melanoma, chemotherapy, radiation treatments, and morphine will not interfere with buying and selling his wares. The ultimate salesman, making "the deal" is John's life.

John's Beliefs about Cancer

John developed what he thought was a plantar's wart in 1973. He treated it with an over-the-counter medication. Liquid fire — salicylic acid — burned out the wart. Fifteen years later this growth re-established itself in the hollow of John's foot; it persisted despite the application of the previous remedy. Concerned about this stubborn growth, John consulted his family physician who referred him to a skin specialist. The dermatologist attempted to treat the growth with nitrogen. This, too, proved unsuccessful. The "wart" grew deeper, fixing solidly to John's inner flesh. Each time the dermatologist applied the killing cold the growth returned. Another more serious form of treatment was needed. The dermatologist prescribed daily formaldehyde soaks for a period of three months.

Well, the way that I used to do it was, the dermatologist said to pour the formaldehyde solution in a saucer, put a sponge in the saucer, and then lay your foot on top so that the sponge would transfer the formaldehyde up to the plantar's wart to try and dry it out.

John asks, "Why would they use something that's so powerfully carcinogenic to treat the plantar's wart?" From John's perspective, the formaldehyde soaks caused his plantar wart to convert to a malignant state. Around the time that John was soaking his foot in these baths, the local media reported the toxic, carcinogenic effects of formaldehyde insulation used in the construction of homes throughout the city. It was a small step of logic for John to connect the cancer-causing properties of formaldehyde insulation with the soak solution.

Well, especially when they're telling us about getting formaldehyde out of the houses and getting it out of insulation and stuff like this. And here a doctor is telling me to treat a plantar's wart with it. Well, it sort of makes me wonder whether there's something wrong there or maybe, maybe the dermatologist wasn't up to date on, on his thinking. He's an older man that works for the clinic.

According to John this plantar's wart was not cancerous until he submerged and dutifully soaked it in the bath. His tone of voice suggests that the physician should have known better. He attempts to make sense of the rationale for the prescribed treatment. Ageism. The dermatologist was "an older man," an elderly physician who was perhaps not up to date on the cancer-causing effects of formaldehyde. John believes incompetence and negligence birthed cancer in his foot.

Convinced the noxious soaks caused his cancer, John writes to a lawyer attempting to establish legal causality. He wants to sue the dermatologist. In his letter, John observes:

The dermatologist prescribed me soaking my instep in a solution of formaldehyde as a method of treatment. I was to put the solution in a pan, put a sponge in the pan, and rest my instep on the sponge. This was to be done a couple of times per day. After repeated treatments this also did not solve the problem. It was after this that I decided to have it surgically removed. Two weeks after the removal the surgeon called and advised that it was MELANOMA CANCER [original in capital letters].

The barrister responds. There is insufficient evidence. Responsibility for the cancer in John's foot cannot be attributed to the dermatologist. While accepting the lawyer's legal opinion, John remains convinced that soaking his foot in formaldehyde was the genesis of his cancer.

Narrative of Suffering: Living with Melanoma

Cancer originated in John's foot. Located in his sole, melanoma invades John's life. It is a mortal wound. As a salesman, John spent a great deal of his life pounding the pavement, walking through the cities and small towns of rural Manitoba, Saskatchewan, and Alberta. John remains a salesman, but he can walk only short distances now, each step a painful reminder of his cancer, of his plight.

Obtaining a cancer diagnosis was serendipitous. John merely sought to free himself of what he thought to be a stubborn planter's wart. It was not a search for cancer. Finding cancer was a matter of pathology policy. All excised flesh is examined for malignancies. In November 1991, the dermatologist who had been treating this wart with formaldehyde soaks cut out the growth under local anaesthetic. When the pathology report came back, it identified the tissue from John's foot as malignant melanoma.

And it's been a lot of worries. Um, um getting your house in order, um, getting wills done and stuff like that, and making sure that everything is looked after. Making sure that my bills are paid on time [nervous chuckle] so that my kids don't have to end up paying anything for me. Cause I haven't worked in the last five years about.

In December 1991, John is admitted to the hospital for extensive surgery to uproot the malignant melanoma. John believed that cutting out the melanoma from the sole of his right foot would cure him of his cancer. "I figured that having the operation, the first operation was going to be the cure-all and unfortunately it wasn't."

A swath of flesh adjacent to the melanoma site is cut away. It is a deadly harvest. The tumour has rooted deeply, growing up into John's foot. Skin, transplanted from his gluteus — the buttock — is grafted to the surgical area, filling the space left by the surgeon's scalpel. John is fine during the first year after his diagnosis. Check-ups are uneventful. Ten months following the operation, however, the oncologist palpates large lumps growing in John's groin. Melanoma lying dormant for a year is now seeding. Pink pits buoyed along by blood seeking fertile ground in John's body. John is admitted for surgery during October 1992. Seed cases, the nodes in John's groin, are surgically removed. This hospitalization lasts 33 days and whatever could go wrong does. Severe infection, a build-up of fluid, and dehiscence at the surgical site — the wound in his groin opens spontaneously — result in an extended hospital stay. John describes his hospital ordeal.

Well, Dr. Y found the lumps in my groin area the first time, the way he found them was through what they call a needle aspiration. And um, they stuck a big needle very deep into my groin area and took some tissue samples and it came back positive and he suggested that I come in and have these lymph nodes removed ... and um, he told me um that it would be about a three-week stay in the hospital and it turned out into a five-week stay because of the, of the stitches breaking and the water retention and drainage problem. And then, of course, the following eight days because of, of infection and water retention.

It is now May 1993 and John undergoes chemotherapy to attack the melanoma growing in his body. According to the oncologist, the chances of a remission are one in five. Realizing his odds, he demands to know how much time he has left to live should the chemotherapy prove ineffective.

The doctor mentioned that there is a one in five chance, you know, of uh, of uh, the chemotherapy being effective. But the thing I wanted to know is now that theoretically it isn't effective, how long have I got left? But I don't think they'll tell me that. Because Dr. Y wouldn't venture a guess either. I asked him the same question. I guess the other thing that I would like to know is where do you go from here? You know, what happens to me from now on? Now that I know that something is going to happen, how is it going to happen? Are they going to have to amputate a leg or are they gonna have to cut me to pieces or whatever? This is all in the dark sort of thing. They don't tell me what's going to happen.

Physicians at the cancer clinic are, from John's perspective, keeping him in the dark. "But what a person would like to know is, if the treatments aren't working, what, what's the outcome gonna be, or what do I prepare myself for?" John wants to know. He wants the physicians to tell him his possible fate. He considers the horrors of melanoma and describes how it might consume him. "Are they going to have to amputate a leg or are they gonna have to cut me to pieces or whatever?" Anxiety in wanting to know the melanoma trajectory. The doctors do not tell John what is going to happen.

I wanted to ask the doctor this question and I didn't. I didn't have a chance. And again I should have written it down. Well, I'm sure that these tumours aren't going to kill me. So what is going to kill me?

John believes the tumours growing throughout his body will not kill him. Discrete hard lumps which he can feel in his groin, his chest, and back — they are just below the surface, skin deep. How could these shallow, painless stones cause death?

John reflects upon his circumstances and upon the future. He cannot plan for the future as he used to. "I don't plan ahead as much as I used to." His future becomes attenuated. Far off horizons become fuzzy and lose their relevancy. Future and past relocate to the present. John wants to know how much time he has left to live. No one tells him directly. He wants a time frame to make decisions about his life and, if the time is short, cutting out the melanoma piece-by-piece is not an option.

Well, Dr. X didn't really explain very much to me. I got more information from my son because of his medical background [paramedic], um, um I guess Dr. X ... sort of explained to me that it was the most deadly form of cancer, uh, however no one will tell me what life expectancy is or either they can't, or won't, or don't think it's, it's a, it's a [strained chuckle] requirement. The reason that I am taking this position [wanting to know about the time remaining] is that if there is a time limit on my living or dying I wish to make use of any time remaining in a quality sense and not being hospitalized or cut up piece-by-piece.

John also wants to know all that he can about his cancer, about his life expectancy. He speaks of quality time. Worried about his mother, John wonders what will happen to her if he dies. According to John, information is something that the physicians do not readily share. "It seems like they only want to tell you as much as they want you to know."

Chemotherapy treatments are discontinued. The lumps do not shrink or soften. Another treatment is tried — radiation. Radiant beams are directed at the cancer during the third week of May with the hope of stopping its growth.

John becomes frustrated with the number of physicians he must consult. Each new treatment results in a change of physicians. John would like to collect the physicians together to answer his questions as a group.

I would like one of these days to have perhaps Dr. A, Dr. B, Dr. C, and this Dr. D or whatever the hell his name is, have all four of them get together at the same time and say, "Now, John, I've done this and I've done this and I've done this now." I want to ask them, "What the hell does it all mean? I've tried all of this now the four of you, what do you suggest?" And I'm sure, I'm sure somebody's going to come up with something. The lumps in here are getting bigger and they're becoming very uncomfortable to walk on. Now does Dr. A [the surgeon] solve that problem or does radiation solve that problem or does uh chemotherapy solve that problem? To the point that when, if this forces me that I can't walk, then I'm going to be a little perturbed. Probably extremely pissed off.

John is desperate for a cure. He assumes the role of a case manager. John knows what needs to be done. He speaks as one of his physicians, "Now, John I've done this and I've done this and I've done this." John's statement has a testimonial flavour; the quest for a cure. John keeps his end of the bargain, his treatment contract. He made an implicit deal with the physicians. He has been a good patient. He has followed the rules. John states, "I've tried all of this now the four of you, what do you suggest?" Gathering all of the physicians together in one room will result in a cure, in action. "And I'm sure, I'm sure somebody's going to come up with something." For John, it is simply a matter of a lack of communication among the physicians. One doctor does not know what the other is doing. The collective wisdom of these specialists has yet to be tapped. John is certain this strategy should result in something positive.

John questions whether the new masses in his groin are cancerous. They may not be tumours, but fluid. One lump located in this area broke open. Once the fluid drained out, the lump resolved on its own. John wants to believe that these growths are fluid-filled nodes. He needs to believe. He must believe.

Would that have been a cyst or would it have been a tumour? Because tumours are actually growths, are they not? So if this was a fluid, what the hell was it down there? Now maybe these other two lumps are fluid too. Nobody's taken a look to find out yet. They didn't do any aspirations on the ones down there. The only aspiration they did was on the one up here. Where they actually took cells. And that's why I question this business. There was three, now one drained, now are the other two, are they capable of being drained?

Draining the remaining two lumps might make them go away. Simply disappear.

John notices a change in his energy level. Priding himself as a "go-getter," this drop in energy bothers him greatly.

Oh yeah, a real drop in energy level. Now whether it's the soreness in the foot and having to limp when I walk and being restricted to the amount that I can walk comfortably, like maybe I can walk two blocks and then I have to sit down and rest. Or, uh, I'll take a pop of that ventolin to get my breath back, but that I don't think is a result of the cancer, that's the result of having chronic bronchitis for smoking for 25 years. That's why I'm low on energy. Can't blame that on cancer. Can't blame that on cancer.

Low energy is the result of 25 years of smoking and chronic bronchitis. John repeats twice, "Can't blame that on cancer." Despite the increasing number and frequency of symptoms, John does not admit that melanoma is the cause of his problems. Truth in his body too terrible to believe.

Visiting Opal

Visiting his mother exhausts John. He slips into a depressed state because of her condition. And yet, he feels the need to have regular contact with his mother, to be good to her and care for her in his own way. It is a classic double bind.

I normally take her a bag of jelly beans and I'd take her candies and I used to do an awful lot of baking at one time and I was taking that down for her and then the home said, "Hey cut it out, it's affecting her diet." Here she's getting all this shit that I'm making for her and she's putting on too much weight and I guess they figured it wasn't healthy for her so they said, "Cease and desist!" When I see her I get very depressed. I'm very depressed. Because I know no matter what I say she doesn't understand what the hell I'm saying. [strained laugh] She wonders what the hell is going on. She doesn't always recognize me. I think that's what hurts the most and a lot of her friends have been out too and they've quit going now because of course she doesn't recognize them either.

Despite his increasing fatigue, John visits his mother four times during the course of his illness. Opal's disease is obvious. She wanders incessantly back and forth up and down the halls. On this visit she recognizes John and offers him a kiss. The recognition is a tender mercy for this son.

John places chocolates in Opal's room, in a dresser drawer. This protects the sweets from others who also wander. Holding her hand they walk to the smoker's lounge where John lights her a cigarette. She quickly forgets and rests it against the couch where it melts an oblong hole in the synthetic fabric. John takes the cigarette from her. Back in

Opal's room, John opens the chocolates. Opal smiles and laughs with childlike delight as the top of the box is lifted; emotions soft as chocolate on a cardboard face. Mother and son walk hand in hand to the front door. John kisses her goodbye. Opal shuffles around and roams down the hall, lost.

John makes his way to the Icelandic Cemetery near Opal's nursing home. An uncle and John's brother are buried there. He is unsure whether a headstone has already been purchased for Opal.

When I did mom's will, we had decided that she would be cremated and she'd be interred in, in the graves in Sandburg. And, there is another thing that I don't even know whether I can decide and if something is gonna happen to me before mom, um, who is going to get around to getting her a gravestone. You know, I should look into that right away because I'm not going to be interred there, uh so I don't have to worry about myself but I should arrange, seeing I've arranged for the funeral already, I should arrange for … I don't know whether Thomas Braden [funeral home] would look after that or not.

It is raining. Low, dark clouds, scud the sky. His head bowed, John limps through the cemetery looking for his family plot. Reading the headstones and searching for familial ground, he wants to find cared-for bones. He is walking to his own grave. He looks up, and smiles. Chiselled into a gravestone are his mother's name and birth date. A lawnmower chipped a corner off the black, flat, stone. John brushes his mother's name with care. Opal has a promised place, a headstone, and John is happy.

Monitoring the Body

John's thick hands carefully move over his body, searching. Lymph nodes swell and surface, snagging his fingertips. In March of 1993, he detects more lumps.

March, hey, I guess in March I noticed that lymph nodes um, um were starting to, one lymph node was starting to develop again and one node had started developing on my chest. And I, I had told my, my surgeon that, you know, I didn't want to spend the rest of my life in the hospital. I didn't want any further surgery and asked him whether chemotherapy could be used and um subsequently I'm treated by Dr. Y. And Dr. Y wanted to start the chemotherapy treatments the same day that I saw him. I found two more on my back now too. Well, I think, maybe a vertebra, it feels out of place right here. It could be anything.

Swellings. Misaligned vertebrae. John lifts his shirt for confirmation of drifting bones along his spine. He observes that the lumps could be anything, but not melanoma. John, however, is frightened.

Betrayal of the body on so many fronts makes it necessary for John to draw a map of these physical insults. His paper and pencil sketch is simple, subjective. He sketches where the numbness and pain reside, where he hurts, and where the new growths are located. CT scans, x-rays, blood counts, and ultrasounds, in contrast are complex, objective measures; official and scientific body facts. Truth in numbers and ghostly grey images. Only John will benefit from his body map. He finds it impossible to remember all his complaints, and uses the map as a memory prompt.

John intends to show his map to the oncologists at the cancer clinic. He wants them to see his suffering. For if they see it they will certainly do something. But no one at the clinic examines John's drawing. Not enough time. Too many patients are slipping beneath the surface.

But like I've noticed a numbness in, in the extremities of my hands and the one foot. But not in the other one, for some strange reason. Okay. So I uh, I'm kinda concerned about that and it's something I'll bring up Monday like when we go for the interview. Then I'm going to draw him a diagram of uh, of my body and where I've noticed changes. Like I've noticed changes up here [his chest], the groin area, there's two nodes now. There were actually three and one seems to have drained and it's gone away. Uh, then I've got another mark on my stomach, I've got another one up here and I've got another one in here. And these are just lumps that I've, I've, I've come across. Now they might be stupid things like sebaceous cysts or something like that but of course I want to know. [uneasy chuckle] Um, so that sort of confuses me a little bit as to how to handle that.

Nodes bud in overwhelming numbers. Melanoma roots in John's lymph system and other sites, growing large and stony hard. Referring to these lumps as "stupid things like sebaceous cysts," John may also be thinking that they are cancerous. These germinations are not painful, yet produce numbness throughout his body. A less palpable but more sinister threat, he loses feeling in the baby fingers on both his hands and in his right leg.

One of the lumps in my groin has become quite uncomfortable when I'm walking because it's enlarged just about double from what it was. It's about the size of a golf ball now.

Loss of sensation and the golfball-sized lymph nodes in his groin make it impossible for John to cross his legs. His right foot swells elephant-like and each foot requires a different shoe size.

The shoe people at the hospital called me yesterday because I was there the day before yesterday and had my foot measured for, because with it swelling I really need two sizes of shoes. I've had to take the, the insole that was made for me, I had to take that out because my foot was swollen too much and I couldn't, couldn't tie the shoe up. Or couldn't get into the shoe and walk comfortably.

John's foot is gruesome. Warm to the touch, bloated, the skin is paper thin. Flesh appears chewed from the instep of his foot, as if an animal had feasted on it. The arch is tender, raw, and open and blood-tinged fluid drains from areas along the sole of his foot. This is where the melanoma first grew; where John's cancer journey began.

John gains weight. Evidence of serious bodily corruption, he inno-cently attributes this weight gain to the tumours growing in his body.

The other thing is I weighed myself this morning and I, according to my scale I've put on just about 18 pounds [over the past month]. And that is unlikely because I haven't changed my eating habits and I'm just wondering whether I'd put on 18 pounds worth of tumours some place as against 18 pounds worth of fat.

Not only has John gained weight, but his abdomen is expanding. He leaves his pants unfastened. Suspenders keep his trousers from falling down. Bending over causes him shortness of breath. He feels as though his breath is being cut short. His belly pushes into his lungs. John searches for an explanation. He believes that not wearing his anti-embolism stockings resulted in a fluid shift causing his abdomen to increase in size.

I wasn't wearing that stocking, now whether that stocking gets rid of the water or not, I don't know. Maybe it just puts the water someplace else. But maybe I should be taking diuretics or something to get rid of the water or something. But nobody's even suggested that.

Despite his deteriorating condition, John attends the flea market. He takes ten typewriters with him and he tries to sell them all. Like the other addictions in his life, John cannot stop being a salesman. His right leg is now twice the size of the left and walking becomes increasingly painful, his limping more pronounced.

It is now the end of July and John can no longer wear tailored pants. He purchases sweat pants, but even these are too small to accommodate his belly. He cuts the sweats and pulls them up over his buttocks. His abdomen is the size of a nine-months pregnant woman's. John cracks open a beer. It is 10 a.m.

Abandonment by the System: The Problem of a Fatal Disease

As John's cancer gradually overtakes his body, the concern offered by nurses and physicians at the clinic wanes visit by visit. Melanoma consumes John. Staff recognize the certainty of his death. Another distancing takes place. Chemotherapy and radiation have failed John at the cellular level and his oncologists cannot save him. John's body speaks of failure. Melanoma grows unabated, tormenting John, taunting his physicians. It thrives in his groin, expands throughout his gut, and interrupts the smooth lines of his chest and back.

But after the doctor did the lymph node, uh, uh, uh, dissection, he never checked anywhere else anymore. He just kept a sort of a check on this and then I mentioned that I had one lump up here and he said, "Then you better come in." But he, he still put me off then and kept me waiting an extra week ... uh, after I had phoned him saying that I had found this lump up here and he said, his nurse said, "Well your appointment's not for two weeks, you come in two weeks time, you know, don't come in any earlier." Cause apparently he was busier than hell and as it was they had to reschedule me.

The staff of the cancer clinic understand the disease trajectory for advanced melanoma. It is a familiar route albeit witnessed from a safe distance. As a lived experience for John, dying is an uncharted voyage.

His is a solitary destiny; a gradual diminishing of the self. John perceives a lack of concern for his welfare at the cancer clinic. Alarmed at the changes in his body he tries obtaining an earlier appointment at the clinic.

He [physician at the cancer clinic] said he just wanted to leave things go. He just wanted to leave things go for two weeks and see whether anything was decreasing in size. He didn't seem to be overly worried about the extra lumps that have been developing. I guess it's just another, the disease is running its course or something. But at least I would suspect that anyway.

John's interaction with another physician at the cancer clinic reinforces his sense of abandonment. The physician's actions convert a general sense of abandonment into a personal experience.

I had an appointment with Dr. X and I tried to ask him some questions and he kept putting me off on the questions, putting me off on the questions. Finally he said, "I'm going to send you down to radiology." And I said, "Just a second, I have some more questions for you." And he said, "I'll be right back," and he never came back. I have three new tumours and I wanted new prescriptions for sleeping pills, I wanted the x-ray results. Find out whether it [cancer] had transferred anywhere else. I wanted to ask him about the experimental drugs, whether he was still using them.

Sensing desertion by the system and the growing remoteness on the part of the care providers, John seeks health care elsewhere.

I'm losing confidence in him [Dr. X] completely. As a matter of fact, I'm going to try to get a hold of Dr. R [personal physician] this week and see if he can refer me to somebody else. I also left two messages with Dr. Y [surgeon] to call me and he never phoned me back.

Angry with how he has been treated, John visits his personal physician who prescribes him a diuretic to help his body rid itself of fluid.

I'm not going to screw around with this [weight gain]. She, she [appointment nurse] gets me an appointment, uh for, for August 10th and I'm worried about this problem now. I figured piss on it. I went uh, I went down to my own doctor who in turn gave me some diuretic pills. I couldn't bend down far enough. I was up to 287 pounds according to my scale and I've been averaging around 260, eh. Now my doctor wants me to take these pills for ten days. You know, uh so it shows me that maybe they're so busy down there [cancer clinic] the right hand doesn't know whether their left hand is uh, is going upwards, downwards, or sideways. I phoned that nurse to specifically tell her about this weight gain, and what should I do about it and she, she phoned back and left a message on my machine saying uh, August the 10th was the earliest she could see me. Well that's bull shit as far as I'm concerned because today is only the 18th of July. So you know, I could die in two weeks or three [uneasy laugh], three weeks. Somebody should be seeing me.

John, in his uneasy laughter and concern with time frames, recognizes his situation as perilous. "I could die in two weeks or three, three weeks." The clinic offers him an appointment in three weeks. There is a sense of panic in John's voice. He has now gained 12 kg in just under two weeks. Somebody should be seeing him.

I didn't give a damn who I see at the clinic. I didn't give a damn who I saw, but uh, I know there's something wrong if you put on 27 pounds in a week and a half. Yeah, you know, something's gotta be wrong somewhere. I think something's kaflooey somewhere, somewhere.

Faith. John loses faith in the clinic. Bloated, his abdominal contents displaced and his stomach compressed by ascites — the fluid in his abdomen — John cannot eat much. His appetite dramatically decreases.

And I, I, last night I brought myself home a Kentucky Fried, you know, just one of the little dinner things. I ate the two buns and uh, and uh, and uh the gravy and that was it. The chicken's still in the fridge. I just haven't had room in my stomach. It's, it's so bloated. My appetite's been nothing, just nothing. Well I've got, my stomach feels full all the time and just hard like a rock.

The Weariness and Fatigue of Cancer

John becomes weary. In June, he reports a profound sense of fatigue. A man who has enjoyed an abundance of energy throughout his life, this dense, leadlike weariness burdens him with a terrible heaviness.

I went out for a drink with Betty yesterday. A friend of mine. She used to
work at the Blue Parrot, she now works at Schneiders. So I don't get to see
her that often so I had two beers with her yesterday morning — well actually
four beers, that's four draft — and was feeling tired, so I came home and
went to bed and stayed in bed all bloody day. I met Betty at 11:00 and by
20 after 12 I was home and by 1:00 I had already had lunch and I was in
bed. And I got up at 1:00 this morning and started working on this thing
and rolling cigarettes for today and trying to get my briefcase half-assed
organized.

He grows more and more exhausted as his disease spreads. "I was
very, very tired yesterday. Well, I've been tired all week." Accompanying this tiredness is pain. John has been taking Tylenol 3 since May.
He has experienced constant pain during the past four months. "I'm
taking Tylenol 3s like they're candy." And now toward the end of June
his pain gets worse.

I'm going to and on the, on the Tylenol 3s I'm going to ask for something
stronger too because I'm having a lot of pain. Especially in the groin area
because that thing [lump] is, is, you know, it's in a position that it hurts
when you walk. And the bottom of my foot is always sore. It's always sore.

From Chemotherapy to Radiation to Morphine

Active treatment options are exhausted. Chemotherapy was discontinued at the end of May. It did not have any significant impact on his
melanoma. Then radiation was tried. Initially, it helped. The beams
shrunk a few tumours and provided John with temporary symptomatic
relief.

Well, he [Dr. Y] was noncommittal but uh ... you know as far as, it sound-
ed like well we're gonna try this last radiation treatment and then he wants
to see me in two weeks so that'll be the week afterwards and if there's any
shrinkage, then he's gonna suggest, by the sounds of it, to continue with the
radiation treatment and if there is no significant shrinkage, then they are
going to have some kind of a meeting and they will decide whether or not
I qualify for any experimental treatment.

The physicians suggest one last assessment of the effectiveness of
the radiation treatment. If it is ineffective they may offer John an exper-

imental, last chance, last hope treatment. The cancer does not respond. It spreads. A stubborn, deadly weed in John's body, the melanoma cannot be killed by poison or by fire. The radiation does not work. The physicians do not offer the experimental treatment to John.

Morphine. John is placed on morphine for comfort, for consolation. It becomes his most compassionate friend. A significant marker in a cancer journey, the morphine offers him surcease.

Uh, they put me on um, on um, on um, on um, on um what the hell do they call it … morphine. They said to be very careful with it. Uh [15 second pause] but it's uh, um … it's slow acting you know, a time release type of thing. And um, so yesterday I slept better than 14 hours and the day before, well since I started taking those on, on, on Tuesday. I've been just sleeping like uh, I came home plunk, and I'm sound asleep.

John is thick with morphine — too much so. His eyes are glazed and distant. For the first time in his life, he sleeps deeply and without interruption. While he is comforted by the morphine, the melanoma grows unabated. He can barely keep track of the pod-like tumours forming throughout his body.

Well, they did x-rays and, then of course I found two more new tu- … two more tumours. One's right here just on the edge of my belly. And one's in the back, three more I found and one more on my tummy here. Still the two in the back, uh two here, one in the back of my neck, a small one in the back of my neck here. So that's 2, 3, 4, 5, 6, 7, 8, 9, 10, 11 now. Eleven that I know of. Now maybe the x-rays showed up some more, I really don't know.

John counts his tumours. He locates them in his body one by one. Collectively, they disclose bodily consumption on a massive scale; uncontrolled, unrelenting growth. The lymph nodes in John's groin become so large that he is again willing to undergo node dissection. He wonders whether his surgeon can remove them.

I think I may stop by and see Dr. Y and ask whether or not this might be able to be removed, just by local anaesthetic. When I, when I mentioned it to uh, to Dr. B, he said he's pretty sure that Dr. Y would say no. But you know, if it makes me feel more comfortable I don't see why they wouldn't do it. Just taking off the pressure. That would make me feel a helluva lot more comfortable.

Granite-hard tumours, buried in his soft flesh, increase in size and number. Soft from years of draft beer, John's belly has now become quarry-like. Flesh to rock.

Draining the Ascites: Resurfacing into the Land of the Living

It is now August and John is admitted to a community hospital. He leaves the cancer clinic behind. Abandonment has come full circle. It is mutual. A surgeon punctures John's gut, draining fluid from his abdomen. The relief is immediate as the pressure dissipates. His belly softens. His spirits soar. Eyes bright blue, his voice strong and filled with laughter, John resurfaces. A reprieve from dying and from suffering. Rebirthed, he moves upward, upward, into the land of the living. Life is sweet and John calls himself a yuppie.

I'm down 17 pounds already, uh, another 2 hours I'll be down another uh, what, another litre. So every 4 hours I'm coming down 2.54 pounds. There's my drain. I just fixed this up myself so that if I decided I wanted to do anything, I'm upward, I'm an upward and mobile yuppie. [laughing] But I just feel so great that, you just can't believe. It's like a new life. It was busy, I got an excellent doctor. He did a very, very thorough examination of me, uh you know, went over the tumours and uh all the little scars and everything and he said, "Well this isn't what the problem is, this is what the problem is so let's work on that first." So then he just left me and I sat around for, oh shit, I must have sat around for an hour and a half, maybe two hours. Next thing you know the nurse says, "Don't go anywhere. Don't go out for a smoke. There's a surgeon coming down to see you." And I said, "A what?" [laughter] And she said, "A surgeon is coming down to see you." So he came in and he said, "There's three ways we can attack this. And it's up to yourself which way you want to do it. We can attack using the way you're doing now which is with the diuretics. Or we can drain it. But draining it is only a temporary thing. Uh, but it might last three months." So I said, "Well shit that's worth it!" And I said, "How long does it take?" And he said, "Oh, not very long." And I said, "Well, when can we get it done?" And he said, "How about 20 minutes?" [laughter] I said, "Let's go!"

This physician is different from those at the cancer clinic, he can do something. The surgeon can solve John's problem in several ways. And moreover, John can choose. The surgeon offers John a 20-minute fix and perhaps three months of comfort. John is ecstatic. For the first time in months he feels great.

And it's just, I just feel great, I just feel great. And I have an awful lot of confidence in the doctor that uh, that looked after me. He's an English doctor, he hasn't been over here very long and, uh, he said there is one other alternative. If you have to go to this business of, of, of, going every three months to come in for two days to have this drained, which you might find a pain in the ass. He said, "I can install a shunt from down here [lower abdomen], where this thing is [drain and bag], up to here, and insert it in something here [subclavian vein]."

The surgeon can "install" a shunt. This operation speaks of permanence and the continued need to redirect fluid from John's abdomen. Draining fluid from his belly was a relatively simple procedure. If necessary, John will undergo this treatment again. He will tolerate surgery to remove a tumour if it blocks a duct. Hope fills him as fluid drains from his belly. John loses a total of 21 kg of fluid before returning home on August 2, 1993.

The Fall: A Narrative of Dying

One week later John falls while stepping off a bus. John, who has shown resistance, who has gone so far along this hard path with its painful treatments, begins a different journey. He falls toward his death.

Oh jeez, I fell when I got off the bus yesterday on my way downtown. The bus driver stopped at a, at an intersection where there's a curb at the front and a driveway at the back and I didn't know that there wasn't a curb there and I stepped down and boom, down I went. I cut myself and bruised myself, but the bus driver came running out. I hope everything is okay. I think that's about the worst of it. I scraped my knee a bit.

John's ascites returns. Internal waters make his abdomen hard and swollen. Changes also occur in his physical appearance. John's girth increases, but his face grows thinner. His cheeks look hollow, sunken. His arms are wasting; stick-like, they are out of scale in relation to his midriff. His skin darkens to a peculiar grey-yellow tinge. His teeth are loose and dirty in his mouth. John is unshaven and dishevelled. Unwashed dishes pile up in the sink. Cups are stacked on his kitchen table and his coffee pot is cold. John sits in darkness. He has not turned on any lights on this dark, rainy morning. He does not care.

Chaos, once confined to his body, erupts in his home and in his life. The melanoma cannot be contained. His cancer grows out of control, consuming John as a person. It is a slow erasure. Morphine, bittersweet, eases his pain but it also contributes to this loss of self. John, beyond reclamation, beyond being saved, enters a downward spiral rooted in physiology. His strength wanes. He can no longer lift his right leg.

You know how I get in the van? Backwards! I, I just got no strength. I got no strength. As a matter of fact I got no strength in my arms either, as a result of it.

Today, the day after his last fall, is John's birthday. John does not receive any birthday wishes. None of his children call him. In anticipation of the calls that might have come, John leaves a message on his answering machine.

And it's my birthday today which reminds me, I've got to change my message on my machine to let them know I won't be home until after 8 p.m.

Thick with morphine, words slur out of his mouth. His eyelids are heavy and he struggles to keep them open, to stay awake. John is agitated, on edge, and confused at times.

Nobody knows nothin. Nobody knows a … damn … thing. I called the cancer clinic, they don't know nothing. Uh … what's her name doesn't know anything, Dr. Y doesn't know anything, so I'm gonna wait until later on this afternoon and then I'm gonna see whether I can find out who the hell do I talk to.

John focuses on gaining information from the cancer clinic. Once again he seeks answers to his hard questions.

Well, basically I asked them, I said, "Lookit, what, what, what's the story about, about changing doctors because it's obvious, if you wanted to put me off for over two weeks and I needed surgery within a week, obviously somebody isn't looking after me." After all of those stupid doctors, and I went through 17 of them, I don't know. It's very frustrating. All I want is some answers. You know, if they give me answers, yes, no, indifferent, uh, I wouldn't give a shit. But this business of saying well we'll have to discuss it with this guy or we'll have to discuss it with that guy or, that, that's a bunch of bullshit as far as I'm concerned. That's crazy. That's absolutely crazy.

John bids on some computer equipment. He cannot stop being a salesman. An act to normalize what is left of his life, it is all he knows. Ascites, fatigue, and weakness render him helpless.

It's so hard to bend over, um … and when I told that um, when I told that, uh, uh, what the hell's her name, uh … [10 second pause], Betty, Betty, yeah. When I told Betty that um, I was getting to the point where you know, I can't tie my shoes, I can't get my stockings on, I can't, I can't do any of these things anymore and I've had three falls this week already.

John falls three more times over a period of two days. He falls to the floor in his apartment and remains there for several hours. He cannot sit up. He is weak.

Three. And that's getting too much. So I think, I think something else should be looked into too. Whether I should be going to physio or because I've got no strength in my legs at all, I've got no strength in my arms, um, um … I've just got no strength anywhere. And I can walk, I can walk like from here to that, to the top of the stairs there and then I sit down and I rest for a bit at a chair up there and uh, then, then once I'm flat on the ground I'm not too bad. I'm thinking of getting one of those emergency call things. Because when I fell on the floor the other morning there, I laid there for two hours before I could get up. I laid on the floor for two hours.

He drops his cigarettes three times in five minutes. One of the cigarettes rolls under the kitchen table making it impossible for John to retrieve it. His coordination is off. Moving a cigarette to his lips takes all his concentration. Previously, his tumours occupied his thoughts — the monitoring and the counting. Counting tumours is less relevant now. Ascites is more of a threat, more central to John's plight.

I haven't, I haven't even looked [at his tumours]. I haven't even looked. That's the least of my worries right now. That's the least, well I shouldn't say it's the least of my worries but … I don't particularly want anymore. I think it, it's this fluid that's draining all my energy. It's just taking it all because Christ, I can hardly move. And not a single doctor seems to be doing anything. And I think they're all confused with each other, to be quite honest. I don't know, maybe a nasty letter to the cancer clinic is the next, next step. Say to hell with it, get [the clinic director] or whatever the hell his name is to look into it.

John believes the physicians are not doing anything. They should be. He thinks that a letter of reprimand might be in order. He will write one. John thinks of Opal and expresses a desire to visit her.

I'd like to try to take mom some stuff and maybe that could be arranged for sometime next week and I don't know how your time is next week. Maybe we could sneak down there for an hour, okay?

John does not write the letter of complaint. No one at the cancer clinic will hear of his plight. John surrenders to his disease. He never sees his mother again.

*

John died three days later in a community hospital on September 10, 1993.

*

Well, my work habits were always based on the premise of "get it done in the morning or don't bother doing it." I've had this work habit as long as I can remember. I would never sleep all goddamn day. My ex-wife, I used to have to fight to get her into bed and fight to get her out of bed [laughter]. I'm working hard these days. I've got about 22 coffee tables that I'm cleaning up and putting wax on them and getting them ready to sell. I got a hell of a lot of work to do, but I'm also aware of the statistics on melanoma. It's only with good luck and by God that I'll live any longer than two to five years, unless anything unforeseen happens.

— John, May 24, 1993

LESSONS LEARNED: JOHN'S GIFTS TO US

Although John's account of cancer is disturbing, we are offered an in-depth understanding of what happened to him. It was only through his story that we were able to briefly walk with him on the consumptive path of malignant melanoma. There were things that John did — and did not do — that contributed to his suffering. Examining the details of his story may spare others the misery he experienced. This is John's gift to us.

Finding Cancer and Receiving a Diagnosis

Like many of us, John made use of over-the-counter medications to treat what he believed to be a plantar's wart. This strategy had proved successful 15 years before when he self-treated a plantar's wart. Despite John's efforts to treat this new growth, it kept returning. John then consulted his family physician who referred him to a dermatologist, who also tried various treatments to remove this stubborn growth on the sole of his foot. Initially, the growth was burned off several times using nitrogen. For another treatment, John placed his foot in a basin of formaldehyde. Finally, the dermatologist cut out the growth under local anaesthetic.

- Sometimes, despite all our efforts and those of our physicians, cancer remains undetected.

- The American Cancer Society has identified seven warning signs that might indicate cancer. It is wise to seek out medical attention if you or a family member or friend experience any of the following:

  - changes in bowel or bladder habits
  - any sore that does not heal
  - unusual bleeding or discharge
  - a lump or thickening in the breast or elsewhere in the body
  - difficulty swallowing or constant indigestion
  - obvious changes in a wart or mole
  - a nagging cough or hoarseness in the voice

- Aggressive, persistent, and stubborn skin growths need to be watched with great caution and checked by a health care provider.

John appropriately consulted his family physician when his self-treatments failed. It was during the dermatologist's third treatment approach — surgical excision — that his malignant growth was finally discovered.

When John was first diagnosed with malignant melanoma, he responded with disbelief and numbness. He cried for several days. He experienced fear and anxiety and asked that profound question of all who suffer: "Why me?"

- Receiving a cancer diagnosis can shake you to the very core of your being. It is not uncommon to experience great fear and anxiety — and for some people, panic. People often respond with shock and a sense of generalized numbness.

- Processing information at this point is often difficult. You need time to integrate your diagnosis. Some people require several days, while others require weeks or months to fathom a cancer diagnosis.

- Because it takes time to assimilate and integrate such a disturbing diagnosis, you may want to consider having a family member or trusted friend accompany you to the initial meetings with your cancer doctor. Although you may listen intently to what your physician tells you, you might not actually hear what he or she is saying about your cancer. Having an extra set of ears can help you recall what the physician said.

- Although a cancer diagnosis may instill a sense of panic or urgency, remember that *you have time to make decisions about treatments.*

- Consider the treatment options available to you. Every choice has a consequence, and you will want to feel comfortable with the decisions you are making.

- After the initial shock of your diagnosis, you may want to find information about your cancer. Facing the unknown is frightening. Finding out about your cancer may make you less frightened.

- A major source of information is the health care team. Your physician, in particular, can answer your questions. Information may reduce the anxiety associated with the uncertainty of your situation and provide you with a sense of control at a point in your life when things may seem out of control.

◆ Your physician, hospital, library, the Internet, and local chapters of the Canadian and American Cancer Societies are good sources of information about cancer and the resources available to you. You can also learn about what resources are available to you in your community from the Cancer Society.

◆ We are spiritual beings and meaning makers. Asking "Why me?" is a profound question and one that people often try to answer for themselves. This question causes us to pause and reflect about our situation in life and our place in the cosmos. Many people try to understand "why" they have developed cancer. Attaching meaning to cancer may lead people to seek out answers from their physician, pastor, rabbi, priest, or spiritual director.

◆ There may be no answer to the question, "Why me?"

◆ For some people diagnosed with cancer, the question becomes, "Why not me?"

◆ Living with cancer is not easy. In your search for meaning, *blaming yourself for your cancer will not help you live with it.* Cancer is a complex disease, the cause of which is not fully understood.

A cancer diagnosis is not automatically a death sentence. John, however, took action regarding his life affairs as soon as he was diagnosed with malignant melanoma. He thought it a good idea to make sure things were settled in his life, just in case. In retrospect, this was a wise decision.

◆ Cancer is not always a fatal disease. If you do not have your life affairs in order, however, receiving a cancer diagnosis should serve as a reminder to have at least a will made out. Make sure that your wishes will be legally respected should you not survive cancer.

◆ Some people establish an "advance directive" to prevent heroic or extraordinary interventions during the latter stages of their disease. Such efforts will provide you with peace of mind. It can also spare your family from further grief.

- Cancer can serve to "push" you to do those things you have been putting off in life. Now is the time to do them.

- Cancer can also serve to urge family members and friends to do those things they have been putting off. Cancer can mobilize people to finally attend to the meaningful things in their lives.

John placed his mother in a nursing home, he wrote out his will, paid all his outstanding accounts, and generally ensured that there were no loose ends regarding his business affairs. We are wise to attend to those things in life that cannot be taken for granted, whether we are diagnosed with cancer or not.

Finding Out about Cancer: The Prognosis

John initially thought that he was cured after the melanoma was removed from his foot. Although he was "clear" for almost a year after his surgery, melanoma resurfaced in his body. People with cancer need to believe that they will be cured and that life can be resumed as it was before the cancer diagnosis. Cancer, however, is a difficult and often unpredictable disease to treat.

- Your cancer is diagnosed based on a number of indicators. Together, these indicators provide an overview as to the nature of your cancer. Your oncologist will know what *stage* your cancer is in. Staging will tell you whether the cancer has spread beyond the original tumour site to other parts of your body.

- Ask your physician about the prognosis (the likely treatment outcome) of your particular situation given the indicators (stage, type of cancer, etc.) associated with your cancer.

- Ask your physician the nature of your treatment. Is the goal of your treatment *cure*? This means that the chances are very good that your cancer will not recur within the next five years. Is the goal of your treatment *long-term management*? This usually means that your cancer cannot be "cured," but managed or treated over a period of several years. If the goal is *comfort care* or *palliative care*, neither cure nor long-term management is possible. This means that your cancer is advanced.

♦ Surgery, chemotherapy, radiation, or other therapies are used to treat cancer. *Treatment failures can and do happen on the cancer path.* A medication may not work on your cancer. If this should happen to you, your physician may recommend a different drug or combination of medications.

♦ Thinking that you are cured and finding out your cancer has spread is devastating. Think positively, be hopeful, but remember that there are no guarantees with cancer.

John's cancer was well advanced by the time he was diagnosed. It had spread beyond the original tumour site. Statistically, his chances of survival were extremely poor. Everyone's body and immune system are different in terms of responding to cancer, and "survival statistics" are based on group data. Applying group data to an individual's cancer experience is not always appropriate or accurate. Although most people might not survive advanced cancer at the time of diagnosis, some do prove the statistics wrong — and live for many years.

People assume that when cancer is surgically removed, they are cured. The intent of the surgical procedure is to remove a malignant tumour from the body. Sometimes this primary tumour site will have "seeded" by the time of the surgery. This is why chemotherapy is sometimes initiated either before surgery or after surgery: to prevent seeding prior to surgery or to kill any cancer cells that have already seeded. John's melanoma was surgically removed from his foot. But the melanoma had already seeded throughout his body, and it eventually took root, grew, and ultimately claimed his life.

Seeking a Second Opinion

John was most uneasy about soaking his foot in a tub of formaldehyde. He had read that formaldehyde insulation was linked to cancer and he wondered if there were risks associated with soaking his foot in this chemical solution. John did not trust his dermatologist and thought this physician was incompetent. Although wary of the formaldehyde soaks, John complied with this treatment over a period of many months. When his cancer was finally diagnosed, John felt that the treatment had caused this wart to become cancerous. Then he wanted to take legal action against the dermatologist.

◆ If a treatment makes you feel uncomfortable or you question the value of it, talk about this with your health care provider. *Do not allow* the medical system to override your "gut" feelings about things.

◆ Your relationship with your physician works best if founded on *trust*. If you do not trust your physician, if you lose confidence in your physician, or if you think that he or she is not providing appropriate care, then you might want to talk with him or her about your perception of the situation. You may consider a referral to another physician.

Seeking out a second opinion might have been beneficial to John. His cancer may not have necessarily been discovered sooner, but he might have developed a more trusting relationship with another physician.

Communicating with Members of the Health Care Team

John wanted to know his chances of survival at several points along his cancer path. He wanted some indication of the amount of time he had left to live. Trying to predict the time left to live is difficult and imprecise. None of his physicians answered John's questions to his satisfaction.

◆ As a person living with cancer, it is your *right* to have all your questions answered.

◆ Let your physician and nurses know if you feel your questions are not being answered as fully as you would like.

◆ If your oncologist continues not to answer your questions, you might consider making an appointment to discuss your questions with the clinic director.

◆ Remember that your family physician can advocate on your behalf. He or she can find answers for you.

◆ Writing out your questions and concerns in advance of your medical appointments is a good idea. Take these lists with you so that you can be focused during your appointment.

- Some people take tape recorders to their medical appointments. It is probably wise to gain permission from your physician to do this. Not all physicians will agree to having their private conversations tape recorded.

John took a body map with him during one of his medical appointments. There were so many things going on with his body that he could not remember everything. This "map" helped him remember his problems and convey this information to his physician. John also wanted to know how he would die. He could not understand how the lumps just below his skin surface could take his life. He viewed these tumours as isolated islands of cancer, self-contained granite stones. John wanted to know what would cause his death; how malignant melanoma might claim his life.

- A wise physician never predicts death. It is often difficult to determine, with any precision, when a person might die. Your physician may be reluctant to provide you with a specific time frame for death.

- Your physicians, however, should be able to tell you "how," in general, the dying trajectory might unfold given your particular circumstances.

- Remember that you have the *right* to engage in these conversations with members of your health care team. Talking with your physician or nurses about *how* your disease might progress may help to alleviate your anxiety.

John asked courageous and difficult questions that were not addressed to his satisfaction. This led him to become frustrated, angry, and resentful.

John's impertinence, his contempt for authority and the system, his abrasive manner and crude language were acts of resistance in his struggle to survive this disease. Because of his temperament, however, John created friction with almost everyone he encountered at the cancer clinic. Trying to survive malignant melanoma placed John in a most vulnerable position. Angered by the perceived lack of concern demonstrated by the physicians and nurses, John burned his bridges with the cancer clinic. He abandoned the clinic as he felt abandoned by the staff. Except for his family physician, this left John essentially without cancer care.

+ Living with cancer can generate emotions such as anger and fear. The uncertainty of this disease can also cause anxiety and frustration. As a vulnerable person who may be experiencing an emotional crisis, you are entitled to care that maintains your *dignity* and is characterized by *respect* and *honesty*. Similarly, those who provide care to you deserve to be treated in a like manner.

+ The sheer number of people providing you with cancer care can be overwhelming. Find out who is responsible for coordinating your care while you are receiving treatment. The physician responsible for your overall care (the physician who coordinates your care) is usually called the attending physician.

John eventually sought assistance from his family physician and finally from a community hospital. John lacked the interpersonal skills to navigate the health care system smoothly. Displaying hostility toward medical and nursing staff sometimes carries a hefty price. In John's case, it led to a distancing between John and the clinic staff.

The Need for Excellent Pain Control

John expressed that he was in pain during the last few months of his life. He was taking Tylenol 3s, but this medication did not appear to adequately manage his pain. He was eventually placed on morphine, but while the morphine controlled his cancer pain, the amount that John was taking "snowed" him. He was too heavily medicated. He could not talk or function adequately in his daily life.

+ Let your physician and nurses know if you experience pain.

+ *Don't wait for pain to get worse before getting help.*

+ Achieving excellent pain control entails an active process during which you and your oncologist work closely together. Your pain medication will likely change over time (the type of medication and/or the dosage), and it may take several tries before you and your physician can achieve pain management with few, if any, side effects.

◆ Good pain control occurs when *you are actively involved* in your care.

John, distanced from the cancer clinic, did not interact with the physicians and nurses. He remained on his own. Consequently, no one monitored how well his pain was managed, nor the side effects he was experiencing.

Cancer as a Lonely Journey

John was profoundly alone on his cancer journey. His personality and life circumstances were such that he lived with cancer on his own. He had limited support from family or friends, and he lost the support of the physicians and nurses at the cancer clinic. Cancer can isolate us from our bodies, ourselves, family, friends, and our community. It takes a real effort to maintain connections with others while living with cancer.

◆ The very nature of cancer is isolating.

◆ You do have a choice of the extent of "aloneness" on your cancer path. If you are alone, and you do not want to be, there are things you can do that will bring people into your life so that you do not journey alone.

◆ If you are alone, ask your physician, nurse, social worker, or spiritual director to "match" you with another person living with cancer. Someone else who is living with cancer may also be in need of companionship and friendship.

◆ You can join a cancer support group and establish new friendships, find understanding, emotional support, and companionship. There are also websites on the Internet where people document their cancer journeys. They invite people to e-mail them and correspond.

◆ There are many cancer resources in your community. Take advantage of what is available for you. Arrangements can be made to have nurses visit you in your home on a regular basis. There are numerous volunteer groups which can offer you support, contact with others, and caring.

John's cancer journey was difficult. The nature of his cancer, malignant melanoma, John's personality, and his life circumstances all contributed to a hard cancer path. Both cancer and John himself contributed to a journey of profound loneliness. In the midst of all that cancer claimed, however, John ensured that his mother was looked after. She was the one person in his life about whom he dearly cared. Despite all the terrible things that happened to John, he directed his energy toward Opal.

John offered us many lessons. His journey revealed that sometimes cancer can be hard to detect and diagnose. Once diagnosed, John thought that his cancer treatment would cure him. We learned from John that there are different goals associated with cancer treatment: cure, long-term management, and comfort care. John was also a gruff and demanding person. His personality caused difficulties for him with respect to communicating with members of the health care team. John's anger and fear alienated him from those who wanted to provide him with health care. His manner left him alone and lonely on his cancer path. It is important to treat those who journey with us with dignity, respect, and honesty. In the shadow of cancer, however, John tried to live as fully as possible. He was a salesman unto his death.

9

CANCER: ON LIFE AND SUFFERING

WE HAVE TRAVELLED a great distance with Julia, Sarah, Madeline, Kay, and John. Each cancer journey reveals a distinct landscape of suffering. Collectively, the five voices chorus the suffering encountered with breast cancer, ovarian cancer, and malignant melanoma. The narratives call out on behalf of those who do not survive their cancer; those who are silenced. Survivors are not the only persons whose stories must be told.

Walking with these five people has also taken us, the observers and the readers, on a journey. Our hearts ached at what happened in these people's lives. We reflected on their circumstances and fate. Reflecting on another's suffering generates empathy and compassion. Getting to know cancer involves fathoming the human condition found in vulnerable, diseased bodies. And to gain some insight into this suffering is also to understand the remarkable resiliency of the human spirit.

Cancer has become socially constructed around the three pillars of coping, hope, and survival. This transmogrification of cancer is revealed in the ideology behind slogans and programs such as "cancer can be beaten," "take control," and "look good, feel good." Cancer patients are expected to live by this ideology. While it may be applicable and acceptable to some, the negative impact of this stance on cancer patients warrants scrutiny. Regardless of outcome, living with cancer is tempered by the reality of suffering. Disparity between the personal experience with cancer (cancer hardships and suffering) and this ideology (coping, hope, and survival) can engender a sense of failure among people. Many of us will walk the cancer path, either directly as persons living with cancer or indirectly as relatives or friends of someone we love who is diagnosed with this disease. This is why the cloak of silence concerning suffering and cancer is potentially harmful. The cancer journey is constituted by more than coping and hope.

Knowing Cancer: Listening to Those Who Journey

Only in the last decade has the "science" of qualitative research received recognition from the biomedical community at large. Qualitative research largely remains undervalued as "subjective" and is considered anecdotal at best by many scientists who adhere strictly to the tenets of the scientific method and true experiments. And yet, qualitative research provides an entrée to the world of persons living with cancer. Qualitative research has the potential to bridge statistical or normative understanding with individual experiences; professional knowledge with personal knowing; and biological facts with social and cultural knowledge. Cancer is not just cells. It is a personal, interpersonal, familial, social, and cultural disease. Understanding cancer necessitates a more holistic research agenda which respects and develops all forms of knowledge.

To date, biomedical researchers have mostly focused on the efficacy of cancer treatments. Efficacy has been determined primarily through evaluation of medical outcomes, years of disease-free survival, mortality, morbidity, and relapse rates.[38] The importance and relevance of this empirical knowing is invaluable. However, it is estimated that almost 75,000 Canadians and Americans die of breast cancer, ovarian cancer and malignant melanoma each year. Beyond the gross efficacy indicators, the *quality of living* for persons diagnosed and treated for cancer warrants serious research attention. Directing research dollars toward improving the quality of life for persons who journey with cancer — and the people who support them — is a moral imperative.

It is only recently that *quality of life* has been recognized by researchers as an important dimension of the cancer journey. However, quality of life research has heavily invested in the quantitative or numerical assessment of physical, psychological, social, and spiritual dimensions of life that are affected by cancer. There is a concomitant need for more qualitative research to understand the intricacies and connections between quality of life issues and suffering.[39] As King et al. observe, "qualitative data contains a wealth of unique insights into the personal stories and dynamic nature of cancer" (37). We are hard pressed to account for cancer journeys; the processes and changes therein. Illness trajectories of persons living with cancer remain relatively unknown. What happens, over time, to women diagnosed with breast cancer? What are the realities of women diagnosed and treated for ovarian cancer? What is the illness trajectory for men and women living with malignant melanoma? How do these cancers unfold within the context of lives?

Women's voices, their encounters with cancer, remain mostly whispers in cancer research. Women's experiences, their everyday lived meanings of cancer, are not well known. This knowledge deficit is recognized by social scientists who are now beginning to direct their energies to the personal and particular experiences of women who journey on the cancer path.[40] The quality of living for women diagnosed and treated for cancer is especially important given the noxious treatment effects associated with cancer, and the fact that thousands of Canadian and American women continue to die of breast and ovarian cancer.

In light of the preceding discussion, how do the five narratives, spanning a period of six months in the lives of terminally ill persons, inform us about cancer, life, and suffering?

Cancer: Suffering within the Context of Lives

The word suffering is derived from the French word *souffre*, which has its origin from the Latin: *sub* [under] and *ferre* [to bear]. At the root of suffering, therefore, is endurance or bearing under. Associated with suffering is a sense of interminability, of unbearable duration and inescapability. Persons who suffer are caught in something that, at the time, seems without escape, without end. Each of the people, whose narratives are chronicled in this book, endured. They could not escape their cancer. Sarah, for example, initially thought she could "outrun" her cancer. She came to realize that she could not. Cancer became an intimate part of their lives.

Cancer itself seemed without end. Treatments (surgery, chemotherapy, radiation) did not guarantee the end of cancer. Even when cancer was cut from their bodies, Julia, Sarah, Madeline, Kay, and John lived with uncertainty and apprehension from check-up to check-up. The fear that cancer on the advance would be discovered was ever present. The journeyers had to learn to live with the uncertainty of cancer.

These five people also had to learn to live with the suffering found on the cancer path, especially suffering rooted in the body. Excellent symptom control of pain, nausea, vomiting, and shortness of breath provides much needed comfort along this path. Medical management of these symptoms is central to living fully while living with cancer. Yet many of these symptoms were not well controlled. Poorly controlled symptoms were a major source of suffering on the five cancer paths.

Each person tried to take action, but sometimes they lacked medical knowledge that could have helped them obtain better care. At other times, they did not feel able to ask questions, or they were incapacitated by their symptoms, and therefore could not take action concerning their suffering. Madeline, Kay, and John, in particular, experienced significant physical pain on their cancer paths. Suffering arising in their bodies consumed much of the energy these people needed for other things — healing and attending to priorities in their lives.

A fundamental characteristic of suffering is the erosion of communication. When we suffer, a distancing between ourselves and others occurs. We draw inward, we focus upon our innermost being at the expense of the world around us. A separation occurs between the individual and his or her world. Paradoxically, in the depths of suffering, people often see themselves as abandoned or forsaken by others. We feel alone. Julia, Sarah, Madeline, Kay, and John all experienced this sense of isolation and aloneness. This is why gently reaching out to those who suffer is so important. Expressing concern reassures those who suffer that they are not alone.

Although people are often aware of others' suffering, they sometimes look away from the plight of sufferers. Many demonstrate what Soelle[41] terms "apathy," a sense of distance from suffering. People can feel uncomfortable encountering this condition in another person. Beyond the individual encounter, our society rejects and tries to ignore suffering. We do not want to know about the realities of a disease like cancer. We want a "quick fix" or at least a self-help manual. We want to hear that "cancer can be beaten." Some dimensions of human suffering are not amenable to such quick fixes. Thus, those who do not suffer often engage in the "look of distance." [42] The din of the world continues, insensible to the suffering of others, to their plight. Auden captures this sense of distance beautifully in his poem "Aux Beau Musée." While Icarus tumbles from the heavens into the green ocean, those who must have witnessed his descent carry on as if nothing amazing has happened; a boy helplessly falls out of the sky. While we suffer, we are surrounded by joy and laughter and the unlimited promises of tomorrow — for others. This can make our suffering all the more painful. It makes us feel even more alone. Something terrible is happening to us and no one seems to notice or care. We feel abandoned as we journey down the cancer path. We are left behind as others continue their life journeys without us.

The five narratives also revealed the following in relation to cancer:

- *The uncertainty of cancer* is a hallmark of the disease. While each person hoped to survive cancer, this hope was undermined by the reality that cancer often seeds. This uncertainty led to a host of fears on the cancer path. In particular, people feared the recurrence of cancer and the dissolution of intimate relationships.

- *Cancer requires courage.* People living with cancer are required to be courageous. Cancer may demand acknowledgement of one's mortality. Courage may also be required of people to speak up and be heard by health care providers. Finding "one's voice" in the cancer experience is itself an act of courage. Talking with authority figures such as physicians can be intimidating. Broaching difficult areas (e.g., treatment failures, palliative care) also demands courage. Many health care practitioners are not receptive to intuitive bodily knowledge and alternative therapies. Addressing these areas means that people who are living with cancer speak up without knowing whether they will be well received by the very people who are providing cancer care. As the narratives revealed, there are also risks and consequences to speaking up and asking questions.

- *Treatment failures can and do occur on the cancer path.* Cautious optimism is a wise stance in relation to cancer. The five people who journeyed with cancer were devastated when they learned of their treatment failures. Such failures can induce an "existential chill." Additionally, some of the people suffered because they were under the impression that their cancer was cured when in reality they were receiving comfort care. There was incongruence between their understanding of treatment and their physicians' treatment plan.

Life and the Work of Suffering

When we suffer, we are forced to submit to and endure a particular set of circumstances. In this sense, we are passive and held captive by our suffering. Cancer occupies the body on its own terms; we are subject to a corporeal invasion, a bodily takeover. Along with the threat to our

body integrity, the integrity of "the self" is threatened. Cassell[43] introduced this idea of personhood and suffering, suggesting that while people suffer they feel as if they are disintegrating. Their personhood
becomes fragmented as they perceive an impending destruction of their
selves. Suffering continues until the threat of disintegration passes, the
integrity of the person is restored, or the suffering is reduced through
the healing of the self.

An active sense of human agency assists people in their suffering
work.[44] As the poet Rilke observes, "*Wie viel ist aufzuleiden*" [How
much suffering there is to live through]. We live through suffering,
even while we suffer. We have the opportunity to be active in our suffering, as a way of healing ourselves through making sense of the suffering and by integrating the losses experienced within our lifeworld.

Often this integration depends upon our living as well as we can
despite the losses and ravages to our body and our personhood. For
example, when cancer caused Madeline to suffer losses of the self,
she tried to adapt to these losses. She underwent reconstructive breast
surgery, she wore a wig when she went outside her home, and she tried
to conserve her energy so that she was well enough to attend church on
Sundays. Being active in our suffering means trying to move forward
with life, even at the same time that loss upon loss accumulates.
Suffering and healing take work.

Suffering may serve as an opportunity for inner growth and change.
Changes in attitudes, relationships, and values are possible through the
work of suffering. Healing through suffering requires an active role on
the part of the sufferer. Healing is also a difficult process that takes us
from shock, through acute distress, to reintegration. It is a process
of creating order out of chaos.[45] Geertz[46] suggested that suffering
occurred when a meaningful life pattern threatened to dissolve into a
chaos of thingless names and nameless things. The order of our universe changes when we suffer. The personal task is to put life back
together again, making sense of what is happening to us, and then
going on from there.

Meaning in the Cancer Experience

Many people try to make sense of their suffering. They situate, or
locate, it within the context of their lives and within the constellation
of their belief systems. Attributing meaning to suffering can sometimes
"tame" it or make it more bearable. We then feel as if we suffer for a

reason. Understanding the reason behind such an assault makes the experience more endurable for many persons. Yet the meaning behind suffering is a uniquely personal determination of the person who suffers. As Cunningham[47] observes:

The search for meaning in cancer, or in any event, is the attempt to place it in its physical, psychological, social, and spiritual context; growing understanding may or may not be accompanied by physical healing, but will bring comfort, an awareness of our connectedness, a lessened fear of death, and a sense of authenticity and purpose in life. (142)

For some people, suffering has a devout and religious meaning. Those with religious beliefs may see their cancer as a test of their faith, as a necessary act of purification, or part of the mystery of God's plan. Suffering may also be perceived as a punishment from God; a state of suffering may mean a state of sinfulness. Or religious persons may view their cancer experience as an opportunity to offer up their pain for others. In this way, the suffering of one may benefit or even spare another. Suffering may be embraced as a means to free a person from the imperfection of human existence and providing a means of coming to God or achieving enlightenment. Although the impact of religious beliefs and spiritual practices on the cancer experience should not be underestimated, George[48] has noted the difficulties experienced by some health care providers who are confronted with the suffering of others:

Physicians need to be interested in the quality of their patients' spiritual and emotional lives, as well as their medical histories, and they need to be open-minded about the impact of religious beliefs and spiritual practices on healing. Being able to hear a patient's deepest fears about dying requires a high degree of spiritual maturity, and it is a rare physician who can be present in such a way. (46)

Meaning of a non-religious nature can occur in the cancer experience. Those who journey with cancer may discover insights into life and the cosmos. For the five journeyers in this book, these were moments of fantastic lucidity. Julia referred to these periods as one of the gifts offered by cancer. She called this phenomenon the "beauty of cancer." She realized that her husband, her children, and her grandchildren deeply loved her. She loved and was loved. Julia discovered the essence of herself and her life as cancer peeled away each layer of herself. Cancer ravaged Sarah's body, but it could not destroy the love that she and her partner shared. She discovered that Andrew loved her beyond anything. She learned of Andrew's abiding love in spite of cancer. In the midst of her cancer and the consumption of her young life Sarah's love for Andrew entered into the realm of the spiritual. Her love for Andrew grew stronger than her cancer. She died knowing profound love.

For some people, there is no meaning associated with their suffering. Their cancer is a profound and intractable experience that cannot be understood within the context of their lives. This can occur with advanced cancer, where suffering becomes a state of being, nothing more and nothing less. John, for example, never voiced meaning about his suffering or where it led him in life. It was something he tried to live through. He attributed a cause to his melanoma, but he did not appear to develop any meaning in his suffering. There was nothing redemptive or restorative in his ordeal with cancer. John lived with cancer, he suffered because of cancer, and he died from cancer.

Living Fully with Cancer

Living with cancer is about much more than surviving this disease. People can survive cancer, but stop living or engaging in life. Living with cancer requires learning to respect it while not permitting it to define us. This resolution is important, given that cancer is often without end in our lives. Julia, Sarah, Madeline, Kay, and John refused to "live cancer," rather, they lived *with* cancer. Cancer remained a part of their lives, but it did not become their lives. They refused to be defined by a disease. Even when cancer ravaged their bodies and unremittingly ate away at their lives, it could not consume everything in their lives.

Accompanying these people as they engaged in some of their activities of daily living revealed suffering as something that was not exotic or that just occurred during crises. There was an ebb and flow to their suffering. Some days were easier or better than others. Some days were unbearable. Suffering during those times could be thick and overwhelming, while at other times it ebbed and abated. For example, at one point, Madeline cried out, "Just let me die." She longed for death. And yet, two weeks later, she enjoyed a coffee and Italian dessert at her favourite café. With her pain controlled, she engaged in life once again. Each person discovered that their cancer had its own rhythm. Vows to "fight cancer" were intermingled with "cancer just defeats me." One person could voice all these perspectives within the span of a few days or several weeks. None of the five cancer paths was smooth or even. Journeys were characterized by emotional and physical peaks and valleys that constantly changed.

The five people who shared their stories wanted to hold onto the "normal" things in life. They tried to grasp the familiar. This was often an elusive goal, especially as their cancers advanced. What they viewed as normal shifted and changed over time. They sometimes bargained with themselves as to what they considered normal: a minute without pain, an hour without fatigue, a day without nausea or vomiting. All debilitating diseases cause an erosion of the self and it is through this loss of self and the meaningful things in life that suffering is generated. Trying to accept or live within the limitations of these "new" selves necessitated the renegotiation of what was normal.

Throughout their suffering, these four women and one man lived as fully as possible. Although cancer threatened their very existence, they focused on living. These people affirmed life and living as often as and whenever they could. This affirmation was not dramatic or heroic. They professed and avowed life in the love they each found in intimate relationships, among family members, and in a higher power. Life was affirmed in the intricate beauty of snowflakes captured and looked at before they melted in the palm of the hand, the promise of life in witnessing the change from one season to the next, and in the boisterous, overhead honking of migrating Canada geese during the fall. It was found in memories and quiet moments. It was felt in the warm touch of another.

Lessons Learned and Gifts Shared

Sometimes suffering cannot be prevented or treated, but must be endured and lived through. Love and meaningful relationships enable us to live with or transcend intractable suffering. It is the love of others, their compassion, empathy and caring, that offers comfort to the sufferer. Meaningful relationships can be with other people, with God or an Ultimate Being, with nature, or with the arts. It is through the connections we make as we journey through life that we can move beyond survival toward living as fully as possible with a consumptive disease like cancer. As Julia observed:

I finally decided that for me, cancer is a touchstone. Touchstone. It's like a point that allows you to identify the values and things that are important to you. A touchstone originally was a black stone that merchants would scratch gold across to see, to decide on the value of the gold or silver, to determine the value of the bullion. I think touchstone describes it best because I have pulled my life across cancer and decided what's valuable. With cancer, we've been given a chance that most people don't get. We're faced with a life-threatening disease and have the opportunity to re-evaluate our lives. And I don't think that most people sit down and evaluate their lives as to what's meaningful and do something about it. I think that the relationships in my life are much more important to me now than a whole lot more of other stuff. You know, I still do my work and I think I do a good job with it, but the relationships in my life are more important.

NOTES

1. Carper, B. (1978). Fundamental patterns of knowing in nursing. *Advances in Nursing Science* 1(1):13-23.
2. Chapman, R., J. Gavrin. (1993). Suffering and its relationship to pain. *Journal of Palliative Care* 9(2):5-13.
3. Gregory, D., J. English. (1994). The myth of control: Suffering in palliative care. *Journal of Palliative Care* 10(2):18-22.
4. Travelbee, J. (1971). *Interpersonal aspects of nursing.* Philadelphia: Davis Publishing.
5. Kleinman, A. (1988). *The illness narratives: Suffering, healing, and the human condition.* New York: Basic Books.
6. Cassell, E. (1991). *The nature of suffering and the goals of medicine.* New York: Oxford University Press.
7. Amato, J. (1990). *Victims and values: A history and a theory of suffering.* Westport, CT: Greenwood.
8. Heidegger, M. (1962). *Being and time.* New York: Harper & Row.
9. Gadamer, G. (1970). *Truth and method.* London: Sheer & Ward.
10. Benner, P. (1984). *From novice to expert: Excellence and power in clinical nursing practice.* Menlo Park, CA: Addison-Wesley.
11. Hortobagyi, G., A. Buzdar. (1995). Current status of adjuvant systemic therapy for primary breast cancer: Progress and controversy. *CA - A Cancer Journal for Clinicians* 45(4):199-226.
12. National Cancer Institute of Canada. (1999). *Canadian cancer statistics, 1999.* Toronto: NCIC, 13.
13. National Cancer Institute of Canada. (1995). *Canadian cancer statistics, 1995.* Toronto: NCIC, 13.
14. Estimate provided by the American Cancer Society's Department of Epidemiology and Statistics. Wingo, P., T. Tong, S. Bolden. (1995). Cancer statistics, 1995. *CA - A Cancer Journal for Clinicians* 45(1):8-30.
15. Petrek, J., A. Holleb. (1995). The foremost cancer — revisited. *CA - A Cancer Journal for Clinicians* 45(4):197-98.
16. Collier, I. (1992). Management of breast disorders: Nursing role. In S. Lewis and I. Collier (eds.), *Medical surgical nursing.* St. Louis: C.V. Mosby, 1379-95.
17. Crane, R. (1994). Breast cancer. In S. Otto (ed.), *Oncology nursing.* (ed.) St. Louis: Mosby-Year Book, 90-129.
18. Bonadonna, G., P. Valagussa, R. Zucali, B. Salvadori. (1995). Primary chemotherapy in surgically resectable breast cancer. *CA - A Cancer Journal for Clinicians* 45(4):227-43.
19. Kinne, D. (1991). The surgical management of primary breast cancer. *CA - A Cancer Journal for Clinicians* 41(2):71-84.
20. National Cancer Institute of Canada. (1995). *Canadian cancer statistics, 1995.* Toronto: NCIC, 9.
21. National Cancer Institute of Canada. (1999). *Canadian cancer statistics, 1999.* Toronto: NCIC, 13.
22. Wingo, P., T. Tong, S. Bolden. (1995). Cancer statistics, 1995. *CA - A Cancer Journal for Clinicians* 45(1):8-30.
23. Clark, J. (1994). Gynecologic cancers. In S. Otto (ed.), *Oncology nursing.* St. Louis: C.V. Mosby, 190-220.
24. National Center for Health Statistics. (1994). *Vital Statistics of the United States, 1991.* Washington, DC: Public Health Service.

25. Wingo, P., T. Tong, S. Bolden. (1995). Cancer statistics, 1995. *CA - A Cancer Journal for Clinicians,* 45(1):8-30.

26. Canadian Cancer Society. (1999). *Facts on Ovarian Cancer.* Toronto: CCS, Publication No. 211479.

27. Clark, J. (1994). Gynecologic cancers. In S. Otto (ed.), *Oncology nursing.* St. Louis: C.V. Mosby, 190-220.

28. Clark, J. (1994). Gynecologic cancers. In S. Otto (ed.), *Oncology nursing.* St. Louis: C.V. Mosby, 190-220.

29. Wingo, P., T. Tong, S. Bolden. (1995). Cancer statistics, 1995. *CA - A Cancer Journal for Clinicians* 45(1):8-30; Clark, J. 1994. Gynecologic cancers. In S. Otto (ed.), *Oncology nursing.* St. Louis: C.V. Mosby, 190-220.

30. Wingo, P., T. Tong, S. Bolden. (1995). Cancer statistics, 1995. *CA - A Cancer Journal for Clinicians* 45(1):8-30; Clark, J. 1994. Gynecologic cancers. In S. Otto (ed.), *Oncology nursing.* St. Louis: C.V. Mosby, 190-220.

31. National Cancer Institute of Canada. (1999). *Canadian cancer statistics, 1999.* Toronto: NCIC, 13.

32. Wingo, P., T. Tong, S. Bolden. (1995). Cancer statistics, 1995. *CA - A Cancer Journal for Clinicians,* 45(1):8-30.

33. Wingo, P., T. Tong, S. Bolden. (1995). Cancer statistics, 1995. *CA - A Cancer Journal for Clinicians,* 45(1):8-30.

34. Wingo, P., T. Tong, S. Bolden. (1995). Cancer statistics, 1995. *CA - A Cancer Journal for Clinicians* 45(1):8-30.

35. Canadian Cancer Society. (1999). *Facts on skin cancer.* Toronto: CCS. Publication No. 211963.

36. Otto, S. (1994). Skin cancers. In S. Otto (ed.), *Oncology nursing.* St. Louis: C.V. Mosby, 361-75.

37. Otto, S. (1994). Skin cancers. In S. Otto (ed.), *Oncology nursing.* St. Louis: C.V. Mosby, 361-75.

38. King, C., M. Haberman, D. Berry, N. Bush, L. Butler, K. Dow, B. Ferrell, M. Grant, D. Gue, P. Hinds, J. Kreuer, G. Padilla, S. Underwood. (1997). Quality of life and the cancer experience: The state-of-the-knowledge. *Oncology Nursing Forum* 24(1): 27-41.

39. King, C., M. Haberman, D. Berry, et al. (1997). Quality of life and the cancer experience: The state-of-the-knowledge. *Oncology Nursing Forum* 24(1): 27-41.

40. Bilodeau, B., L. Degner. (1996). Information needs, sources of information, and decisional roles in women with breast cancer. *Oncology Nursing Forum* 23(4):691-96; Carter, B. (1997). Women's experiences of lymphedema. *Oncology Nursing Forum* 24(5):875-82; Chalmers, K., K. Luker. (1996). Breast self-care practices in women with primary relatives with breast cancer. *Journal of Advanced Nursing* 23(6):1212-20; Dow, K., B. Ferrell, S. Leigh, J. Ly, P. Gulasekaram. (1996). An evaluation of the quality of life among long-term survivors of breast cancer. *Breast Cancer Research and Treatment* 39(3):261-73; Degner, L., L. Kristjanson, D. Bowman, et al. (1997). Information needs and decisional preferences in women with breast cancer. *Journal of the American Medical Association* 227(18):1485-92.

41. Soelle, D. (1975). *On suffering.* New York: Harper & Row.

42. Slatoff, W. (1985). *The look of distance: Reflections on suffering and sympathy in modern literature — Auden to Agee, Whitman to Woolf.* Columbus: Ohio State University Press.

43. Cassell, E. (1991). *The nature of suffering and the goals of medicine.* New York: Oxford University Press.

44. The concept of the "work of suffering" is attributed to Mark Nichter, Department of Anthropology, University of Arizona. Nichter, M. (1990). *On alchemy of work and the lessons gained from the witnessing of suffering in other lifeworlds.* Speech given at the American Anthropological Association Meeting, New Orleans.

45. Kleinman, A. (1988). The personal and social meaning of illness. In A. Kleinman (ed.), *The illness narratives: Suffering, healing and the human condition.* New York: Basic Books, 31-55.

46. Geertz, C. (1966). Religion as a cultural system. In M. Benton (ed.), *Anthropological approaches to the study of religion.* London: Tavistock, 1-46.

47. Cunningham, A. (1992). *The healing journey: Overcoming the crisis of cancer.* Toronto: Key Porter Books.

48. George, P. (1996). A call for open mindedness. *Minnesota Medicine* 79(12):10, 11, 46.